Data Set Directory of Social Determinants of Health at the Local Level

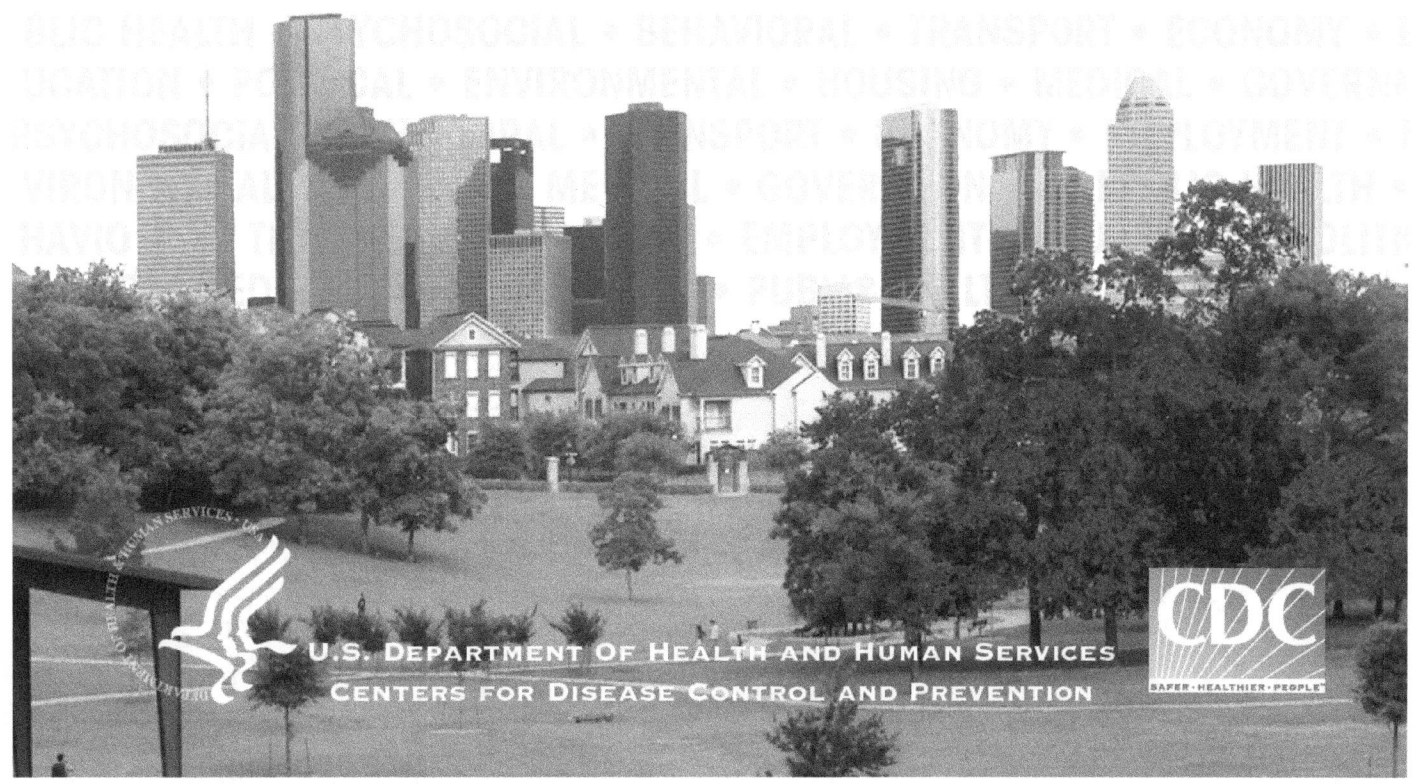

U.S. DEPARTMENT OF HEALTH AND HUMAN SERVICES
CENTERS FOR DISEASE CONTROL AND PREVENTION

CDC
SAFER·HEALTHIER·PEOPLE™

Suggested Citation
Hillemeier M, Lynch J, Harper S, Casper M. Data Set Directory of Social Determinants of Health at the Local Level. Atlanta: U.S. Department of Health and Human Services, Centers for Disease Control and Prevention; 2004.

For More Information
E-mail: ccdinfo@cdc.gov
Write: National Center for Chronic Disease Prevention and Health Promotion
            Division of Adult and Community Health
            Cardiovascular Health Branch
            4770 Buford Highway NE
            MS K-47
            Atlanta, GA 30341-3717

Online
This publication is available at http://www.cdc.gov/cvh.

Acknowledgements
The authors would like to thank the following people for their valuable contributions to the publication of this directory: the workshop participants (listed on page iii) for providing their expert opinions on the dimensions and components of the social environment; Kurt Greenlund and Ishmael Williams for their involvement in the early stages of this project; Mark Harrison for the beautiful cover design, his expertise in formatting information-rich tables, and his great editorial skills; and Amanda Crowell for serving as an excellent copy editor.

This work was funded by ASPH/CDC/ATSDR Cooperative Agreement S1091-19/19.

Data Set Directory of Social Determinants of Health at the Local Level

Marianne Hillemeier, PhD
Pennsylvania State University

John Lynch, PhD
University of Michigan

Sam Harper, MSPH
Centers for Disease Control and Prevention

Michele Casper, PhD
Centers for Disease Control and Prevention

The contents of this directory are adapted from the following article: Hillemeier M.M., J. Lynch, S. Harper, and M. Casper. 2003. "Measuring contextual characteristics for community health." Health Services Research 38(6 part 2):1645-717.

This document is published in partnership with the Social Determinants of Health Work Group at the Centers for Disease Control and Prevention, U.S. Department of Health and Human Services

Workshop Participants[*]

Donna Armstrong
University at Albany, SUNY
Department of Epidemiology

Elizabeth Barnett
West Virginia University
Department of Community Medicine

Stuart Batterman
University of Michigan
Environmental Health Sciences

Matt Boulton
Michigan Department of Community Health
Bureau of Epidemiology

Michele Casper
Centers for Disease Control and Prevention
Cardiovascular Health Branch

George Davey Smith
University of Bristol
Department of Social Medicine

Allen Dearry
National Institute of Environmental
    Health Sciences

Ana Diez Roux
Columbia University
Division of General Medicine

Jim Dunn
University of British Columbia
Department of Health Care and
    Epidemiology

Bonnie Duran
University of New Mexico School
    of Medicine
Department of Family and Community
    Medicine

Anne Ellaway
University of Glasgow
Social and Public Health Sciences Unit

Arline Geronimus
University of Michigan
Department of Health Behavior and Health
    Education

Kurt Greenlund
Centers for Disease Control and Prevention
Cardiovascular Health Branch

Sam Harper
National Center for Health Statistics, CDC
Office of Analysis, Epidemiology and
    Health Promotion

Marianne Hillemeier
Pennsylvania State University
Department of Health Policy and
    Administration

James House
University of Michigan
Survey Research Center

George Kaplan
University of Michigan
Department of Epidemiology

James Krieger
Epidemiology Planning and Evaluation
Public Health–Seattle and King County

Nancy Krieger
Harvard School of Public Health
Department of Health and Social Behavior

Verna Lamar-Welch
Centers for Disease Control and Prevention
Cardiovascular Health Branch

Tama Leventhal
Teachers College, Columbia University
Center for Children and Families

Cynthia Lopez
University of New Mexico School of Medicine
Department of Family and Community Medicine

John Lynch
University of Michigan
Department of Epidemiology

Jeffrey Morenoff
University of Michigan
Department of Sociology

Patricia O'Campo
Johns Hopkins University
School of Hygiene and Public Health

Elsie Pamuk
National Center for Health Statistics, CDC
Office of Analysis, Epidemiology, and
    Health Promotion

Harold Pollack
University of Michigan,
Department of Health Management
    and Policy

Amy Schulz
University of Michigan
Department of Health Behavior and
    Health Education

Mary Shaw
University of Bristol
School of Geographical Sciences

Sharon Simonton
University of Michigan
Department of Epidemiology

Mah-jabeen Soobader
Rochester General Hospital
Division of General Pediatrics

Gavin Turrell
Queensland University of Technology
School of Public Health

Norman Waitzman
University of Utah
Department of Economics

Pamela Waterman
Harvard School of Public Health

David Williams
University of Michigan
Survey Research Center

Ishmael Williams
Centers for Disease Control and Prevention
Cardiovascular Health Branch

Doug Willms
University of New Brunswick
Faculty of Education

John Wooding
University of Massachusetts, Lowell
Regional Economic and Social Development

Michael Woolcock
World Bank

Contents

Continued on next page

Contents, Continued

Introduction to the Data Set Directory

There is widespread interest in the role of local social determinants of health at the local level. Federal, state, and local government agencies, academic institutions, and community organizations are increasingly recognizing the need to understand and address the socioeconomic contexts within which people work and play in order to improve their health and welfare. There is renewed emphasis on implementing interventions aimed at improving socioenvironmental conditions. Such interventions have the potential to produce wide-ranging health benefits (see the April 2003 supplement of the *American Journal of Preventive Medicine*) and could reduce marked health disparities that remain a high-priority concern for public health (USDHHS 2000). It is critical that decisions regarding how to improve health and eliminate health disparities are integrated into the larger picture of community characteristics that promote or endanger health. A recent theme in the literature and in meetings of interested parties around the country is the need for improved conceptualization and availability of data on how the social environment impacts the health of populations (Pickett and Pearl 2001; Macintyre and Ellaway and Cummins 2002; Yen and Syme 1999; Kaplan and Lynch 1997, 2001; Diez Roux 2004; Berkman 2004; Krieger and Davey Smith 2004; Institute of Medicine 1997; M. Miringoff and M.L. Miringoff 1999; Howell et al. 2003).

This *Data Set Directory of Social Determinants of Health at the Local Level* is a response to those needs. The directory contains an extensive list of existing data sets that can be used to address these determinants. The data sets are organized according to 12 dimensions, or broad categories, of the social environment. Each dimension is subdivided into various components.

This directory grew out of a project based at the University of Michigan School of Public Health and funded by the Centers for Disease Control and Prevention (CDC). Investigators from the United States and Europe were invited to a workshop to review an initial list of dimensions important for understanding social determinants of health. Participants represented a wide range of disciplines including epidemiology, sociology, geography, medicine, demography, economics, developmental psychology, education, and toxicology. Others with interests and expertise in the effects of community contextual characteristics on health were also invited, including government experts on data sources and geographic information systems, public health practitioners, and experts on community consultation and processes.

Continued on next page

Structured discussions among the workshop participants led to consensus on a core set of 12 dimensions. Participants then generated detailed lists of components within each dimension, along with suggestions for possible data sources and specific variables that might be used to measure the components of each dimension. Based on the results of the workshop, the lists of components and data indicators were refined by the University of Michigan staff, taking into consideration both conceptual relevance and availability of appropriate data at the local level. An extensive search for data sets that address each of the dimensions and components was conducted–including both traditional and non-traditional sources. The results of this search are presented in this directory.

We focused primarily, but not exclusively, on data sets that contain information for Metropolitan Statistical Areas (MSAs). We chose to focus on MSAs primarily because there is a broad range of data for MSAs that is routinely collected and geocoded. We recognize, however, that there is no single ideal level for measuring social determinants of health in relationship to health-damaging and health-promoting factors. In fact, different characteristics may operate at different levels. An argument can be made that using more localized units, such as county, zip code, census tract, and census block, increases the likelihood of measuring certain aspects of the social and physical environment actually experienced by individuals. Conversely, considerably more richly detailed contextual data sources are available for larger units such as states. Given the inevitable trade-offs between data availability and proximity to lived experience, we chose to focus on MSAs.

Dimensions of the Social Environment

This table lists the 12 dimensions of the social environment.

Each section begins with a brief overview of the literature for each dimension. These reviews are not exhaustive, but rather provide some of the background that led to them being included in this directory.

Each dimension is divided into several components. Each component has one or more indicators, and for each indicator at least one data set is listed.

Economy

Overview

The association between higher levels of economic resources and more optimal health is one of the most well-documented relationships in public health research (Susser and Watson and Hopper 1985; Krieger et al. 1993; Lynch and Kaplan 2000), and economic aspects of local areas have been among the most frequently analyzed contextual factors with regard to mortality and other outcomes. Significant associations have been shown between health status and community economic characteristics including income (Anderson et al. 1997; Diez Roux et al. 1997) and inequality in income distribution (Lynch et al. 1998; Kennedy et al. 1998), wealth (Diez Roux et al. 1997; O'Campo et al. 1997), poverty (Yen and Kaplan 1999; Shaw et al. 2000), and the geographic concentration of poverty (Waitzman and Smith 1998a,b).

The fact that data for most of these economic indicators are readily available for small areas in census data is undoubtedly an important factor accounting for their widespread use (Mitchell et al. 2000). Our consultants encouraged a broadened perspective to more fully assess the economic status of communities. On one hand, this involved identifying a more diversified set of indicators for commonly studied components, such as considering various types of income (earnings, investments, and transfers) in addition to the overall mean or median income in an area. On the other hand, a number of additional components of economic well-being were also suggested for inclusion. For example, the opportunities for community residents to obtain financial resources would be influenced by characteristics of economic development in an area, including productivity, industrial mix, and amount of area business lending, as well as by the exchanges of goods and services through the informal economy. The availability of financial services such as banks and other sources of credit were considered important, as were local costs of living, patterns of redistribution through taxes and transfers, and the fiscal capacity of the area. One other seldom-considered aspect of the economic milieu concerns the degree to which segments of the community are differentially exploited, and thereby constrained in their access to monetary resources. Indicators of exploitation include the ratio of wages to corporate profits, as well as issues related to location of jobs such as length of commute and commuter taxation.

4

Economy Data Sets

This table presents the components and indicators of the economic dimension. Nine economic components are identified:

1. Income
2. Wealth
3. Poverty
4. Economic Development
5. Financial Services
6. Cost of Living
7. Redistribution
8. Fiscal Capacity
9. Exploitation

Within each component, several indicators are identified, and for each indicator at least one data set is listed.

Components and Indicators	Data Sources and Notes
1. Income	
A. Earned income	
1. Median and per capita annual income	Census Bureau (www.census.gov).
2. Mean hourly and annual wage	Bureau of Labor Statistics (stat.bls.gov/oes/home.htm). Data by occupation available in downloadable Excel files.
3. Hourly wage, union, and nonunion workers	Union Membership and Earnings Data Book (www.bna.com/bnaplus/labor/laborrpts html). Separate tables for public and private sector workers and for manufacturing and nonmanufacturing workers. Customized reports available for any or all years since 1983.
4. Per capita personal income	Bureau of Economic Analysis (www.bea.doc.gov/bea/regional/reis). Downloadable compressed comma-separated-value files.
B. Disposable income	
1. Median and per capita Effective Buying Index	Demographics U.S.A (www.tradedimensions.com/p_demographics html). Effective Buying Index represents money income minus taxes. Data available on CD-ROM.
C. Income distribution	
1. Gini coefficient of income inequality; 90%ile/10%ile ratio	Census Bureau (www.census.gov).

Continued on next page

Economy Data Sets, Continued

Components and Indicators	Data Sources and Notes
1. Income (continued)	
D. Geographic concentration of income	
1. Concentration of poverty...........................	Jargowsky, P. A. 2003. Stunning Progress, Hidden Problems: The Dramatic Decline of Concentrated Poverty in the 1990s (www.brookings.edu/dybdocroot/ es/urban/publications/jargowskypoverty.pdf). Percentage of the poor residing in high poverty neighborhoods; total and race-specific rates.
E. Economic segregation	
1. Dissimilarity index (d), poor/nonpoor segregation; Contact index (xPy*), poor/nonpoor segregation........................	Sociometrics Contextual Data Archive (www.socio.com). Downloadable compressed data files for PC and UNIX, including raw data and SPSS and SAS files.
2. Wealth	
A. Geographic concentration of wealth	
1. Mean and median net worth	ESRI Business Information Solution (www.esribis.com). Data can be integrated into ArcGIS.
B. Debt levels	
1. Bankruptcy filings	Economy.com (www.economy.com/research). Personal and business bankruptcy filings and rates per thousand households, by type.
C. Savings rates	
1. Dollar amount of deposits in savings institutions and banks	Federal Deposit Insurance Corporation (www3 fdic.gov/sod/index.asp). From Web site page, choose Summary Tables, then MSA or county tables.
D. Real estate ownership/values	
1. Median value owner-occupied housing units.....	Census Bureau (www.census.gov).
3. Poverty	
A. Geographic concentration of poverty	
1. Poverty rate...	Census Bureau (www.census.gov).
2. Concentration of poverty.......................	See Jargowsky 2003.
B. Deprivation associated with poverty-level income	
1. Percent of families with incomes less than half of the poverty line.............................	Census Bureau (www.census.gov).

Continued on next page

Economy Data Sets, Continued

Components and Indicators	Data Sources and Notes
4. Economic Development	
A. Productivity	
1. Gross metropolitan product (GMP) and GMP growth rate..	U.S. Metro Economies (usmayors.org/uscm/home.asp). Downloadable tables in PDF.
B. Industrial mix	
1. Wholesale, retail, service, and manufacturing establishments...	Census Bureau, Economic Census (www.census.gov).
C. Business lending indicators	
1. City governments bond ratings............................	Statistical Abstract of the United States (www.census.gov/statab/www). From this Web site page, select desired year; select State and Local Government Finances and Employment.
5. Financial Services	
A. Availability of credit	
1. Home loan denial rates by race, applicants with incomes <50%, 50-79%, 80-99%, 100-119%, and ≥120% of MSA median	Federal Financial Institutions Examination Council, Home Mortgage Disclosure Act data (www ffiec.gov/reports htm). From this Web site page, choose Aggregates Reports under Home Mortgage Disclosure Act; select state and MSA of interest; Aggregate Table 5-2 Disposition of applications for conventional home purchase loans, by income and race of applicant, is downloadable as PDF or spreadsheet.
B. Availability of banking and check-cashing services	
1. Number of bank and savings institution offices	Federal Deposit Insurance Corporation (www3 fdic.gov/sod/index.asp). From this Web site page, choose Summary Tables, then MSA or county tables.
6. Cost of Living	
A. Local cost of living indices	
1. Cost of living index: composite/grocery items/housing/utilities/transportation/health care; average local prices for a wide range of specific food items, products, and services	American Chamber of Commerce Researchers Association (www.accra.org). Quarterly and annual average data may be purchased as downloadable spreadsheet or hardcopy.

Continued on next page

Economy Data Sets, Continued

Components and Indicators	Data Sources and Notes
6. Cost of Living (continued)	
A. Local cost of living indices (continued)	
2. Basic family budget: total/housing/food/child care/health care/transportation/taxes	Economic Policy Institute: Hardships in America (epinet.org). From this Web site page, choose Basic Family Budget Calculator; select a metropolitan area of interest or download budget tables for all areas in Excel.
B. Spending/consumption patterns	
1. Consumer expenditures: total/food/alcoholic beverages/housing/apparel/transportation/ health care/entertainment/personal care products and services/reading/education/ tobacco products/personal insurance and pensions	Bureau of Labor Statistics (BLS) (www.bls.gov). From this Web site page, select Consumer Expenditures; select Tables Created by BLS; select current MSA tables grouped by region in text format or PDF.
C. Income to spending ratios	
1. Ratio annual income/expenditures	Can be calculated from BLS expenditures data.
7. Redistribution	
A. Taxes	
1. Local tax rates..	1. Statistical Abstract of the United States (www.census.gov/statab/www). From this Web site page, select desired year; select State and Local Government Finances and Employment.
	2. Tax Foundation (www.taxfoundation.org). From this Web site page, select State Finance; select Combined State and Local Tax Burdens as a Percentage of Income, by State.
2. Cigarette tax	Tax Foundation (www.taxfoundation.org). From this Web site page, select State Finance; select Various Tax Rates.
3. Taxpayers filing for Earned Income Tax Credit	Brookings Institution (www.brook.edu/es/urban/eitc/eitcnational.pdf).
B. Transfers	
1. Transfer payments...	Bureau of Economic Analysis (www.bea.doc.gov/bea/regional/reis). Downloadable compressed comma-separated-value files.

Continued on next page

Economy Data Sets, Continued

Components and Indicators	Data Sources and Notes
8. Fiscal Capacity	
A. Property values	
1. Median value, owner-occupied housing units....	Census Bureau (www.census.gov).
B. Sales levels	
1. Dollar amount of retail sales per household.......	1. Demographics USA (tradedimensions.com/p_demographics html). Data available on CD-ROM. 2. State and Metropolitan Area Data Book (www.census.gov/statab/www/smadb.html).
C. Income capacity	
1. Buying power index	Demographics USA (www.tradedimensions.com/p_demographics html). A weighted index incorporating population, economic, and distributional information to measure the market's ability to buy, expressed as a percentage of the national total (100%). Data available on CD-ROM.
2. Standardized fiscal health................................	State of the Nations Cities Database (policy.rutgers.edu/cupr/sonc/sonc htm). Defined by Ladd and Yinger (America's Ailing Cities: Fiscal Health and the Design of Urban Policy. Baltimore: Johns Hopkins University Press. 1991) as the difference between a city's revenue-raising capacity and its expenditure need expressed as a percentage of capacity. Used to reveal the net effect of a city's economic, social, and demographic characteristics on a city's ability to deliver a standard level of public services at a standard tax burden on its residents. Database available in four PC formats (tab-delimited ASCII, SPSS portable, Excel, and SAS) and one Macintosh format.

Continued on next page

Social Determinants of Health at the Local Level

Economy Data Sets, Continued

Components and Indicators	Data Sources and Notes
9. Exploitation	
A. Ratio of wages to corporate profits	
1. Ratio of average production worker wage: average value added per manufacturing employee...............................	Can be calculated from data in State and Metropolitan Area Data Book 1991 (www.census.gov/statab/www/smadb html).
2. Ratio of average nonunion worker wage: average union worker wage...............................	Can be calculated from data in the Union Membership and Earnings Data Book (www.bna.com/bnaplus/labor/laborrpts html).
B. Commuter taxes	
1. Transit and vanpool tax exemption benefits	Federal Transit Administration (www fta.dot.gov/library/policy/cc/tvbtei.html). Data on which states allow federally exempted, qualified transportation fringe benefits to be exempted from state tax.
C. Commuting patterns	
1. Means of travel to work; median travel time to work; median income by means of transport to work; median income and number of workers in household by vehicles available.....................	Census Bureau, Transportation Planning Package (www.census.gov).
2. Travel time index...............................	Texas Transportation Institute (mobility.tamu.edu/). Annual Urban Mobility Report includes a Travel Time Index, reflecting the average amount of extra time it takes to travel in the peak period relative to free-flow travel.

Employment

Overview

Aspects of employment in residential areas have also been among the more frequently considered factors in research on context and health. Adverse outcomes have generally been found to be positively associated with higher community levels of unemployment (Guest and Almgren and Hussey 1998; LeClere and Rogers and Peters 1998), as well as with larger proportions of employed residents working at lower social class occupations (Armstrong et al. 1998; Cubbin and LeClere and Smith 2000). Unemployment rates and/or occupational status measures are also frequently combined with other indicators of areal deprivation, including median income, car ownership, education level, and overcrowded housing, to form summary measures that are associated with poorer health (e.g., Townsend and Phillimore and Beattie 1988; Carstairs and Morris 1989).

In addition to the usual employment indicators, we include a number of other measures. Looking in detail at characteristics of the workforce, for example, along with the area business capacity and the geography of job growth would facilitate assessment of job access, as well as the degree of spatial "mismatch," which may adversely affect the employment opportunities of central city residents (Holzer 1991; Mouw 2000). Racial, gender-based, and anti-gay discrimination also limit access to employment and can cause stress-related consequences for health (Williams 1999; Krieger and Sidney 1997; Yen et al. 1999). The degree to which occupational safety regulations and policies are in place and enforced is likely to influence the frequency and severity of work-related injuries (McQuiston and Zakocs and Loomis 1998), while aspects of job quality, including wage equity, family-friendly policies, and demand/control characteristics of jobs, can reduce or exacerbate job-related stress and its sequelae (Cheng et al. 2000; de Jonge et al. 2000; A. L. Saltzstein and Ting and G.H. Saltzstein 2001). The presence of labor unions is also associated with more optimal working conditions and employee compensation (Hirsch and Macpherson 2001).

Employment Data Sets

This table describes the components and indicators of the employment dimension. Seven employment components are identified:
1. Employment/Unemployment Rates
2. Workforce Characteristics
3. Area Business Capacity
4. Job Access
5. Occupational Safety
6. Job Quality
7. Job Characteristics
Within each component, several indicators are identified, and for each indicator at least one data set is listed.

Components and Indicators	Data Sources and Notes
1. Employment/Unemployment Rates	
A. Job security	
1. Employment volatility	State of the Nation's Cities Database (policy rutgers.edu/cupr/sonc/sonc.htm). Variables calculated by the Center for Urban Policy Research for this database indicating employment volatility relative to volatility in the United States as a whole. Database available in four PC formats (tab-delimited ASCII, SPSS portable, Excel, and SAS) and one Macintosh format.
B. Labor market turnover	
1. Unemployment rates: total, by race/ethnicity, sex, occupation, and industry	1. Bureau of Labor Statistics, Local Area Series (stats.bls.gov/lau/). From this Web site page, select monthly or annual average tables of total unemployment rates for metropolitan areas; tables available in PDF.
	2. Bureau of Labor Statistics, Geographic Profile Series (stats.bls.gov/opub/gp/laugp htm). From this Web site page, select Estimates for Metropolitan Areas and Cities; tables available in PDF.
2. Labor force participation rates: total, by race/ethnicity and sex	Bureau of Labor Statistics, Geographic Profile Series (stats.bls.gov/opub/gp/laugp htm). From this Web site page, select Estimates for Metropolitan Areas and Cities.

Continued on next page

Employment Data Sets, Continued

Components and Indicators	Data Sources and Notes
2. Workforce Characteristics	
A. Racial/ethnic/gender diversity	
1. Percent distribution of employed persons by sex, race/ethnicity, and occupation..............	Bureau of Labor Statistics, Geographic Profile Series (stats.bls.gov/opub/gp/laugp htm). From this Web site page, select Estimates for Metropolitan Areas and Cities.
2. Percent of workers who are female	Union Membership and Earnings Data Book (www.bna.com/bnaplus/labor/laborrpts.html). Total, private, public sector, and private manufacturing workers; customized reports available for any or all years since 1983.
B. Skill level	
1. Percent distribution of employed persons by sex, race/ethnicity, and occupation..............	Bureau of Labor Statistics, Geographic Profile Series (stats.bls.gov/opub/gp/laugp htm).
C. Unionization	
1. Percent of workforce unionized; percent of workers covered by union contract	Union Membership and Earnings Data Book (www.bna.com/bnaplus/labor/laborrpts.html). Total, private, public sector, and private manufacturing workers; customized reports available for any or all years since 1983.
2. Collective bargaining protection laws covering state and local employees; laws protecting public employees' right to strike	Dilts, D. A., C. R. Deitsch, and A. Rassuli. 1992. Labor Relations Law in State and Local Government. Westport, CT: Quorum Books.
3. Area Business Capacity	
A. Tax breaks offered	
1. Corporate income tax rate	Tax Foundation (www.taxfoundation.org). From this Web site page, select State Finance; select Corporate Income Tax Rates.
B. Number and size of businesses	
1. Number of establishments by employment size (1-4, 5-9, 10-19, 20-49, 50-99, 100-249, 250-499, 500-999, ≥1,000 employees)..........	County Business Patterns (www.census.gov/pub/epcd/cbp/download/cbpdownload html). Downloadable comma-delimited data files and record layout documentation.
C. Business space available	
1. Commercial office space (sq ft) in and outside central business district.....................	Society of Industrial and Office Realtors (www.sior.com). From this Web site page, select Publications; online data from Comparative Statistics of Industrial and Office Real Estate Markets available for purchase.
2. Commercial office space vacancy rate in and outside central business district	Society of Industrial and Office Realtors (www.sior.com).

Continued on next page

13

Employment Data Sets, Continued

Components and Indicators	Data Sources and Notes
4. Job Access	
A. Geography of job growth	
1. Central city and suburban: employment growth rate; number and percent change in number of jobs; share and percent change in share of private employment	Brookings Institution. Brennan J., and E.W. Hill. 1999. Where Are the Jobs? Cities Suburbs, and the Competition for Employment (www.brook.edu/es/urban/hillfa.pdf).
2. Number and increase in nonagricultural jobs	Blue Chip Job Growth Update: Arizona State University (www.cob.asu.edu/seid/eoc/pubs/JGUsample). From this Web site page, select Ranking of MSAs.
B. Discrimination/affirmative action policies	
1. Employment-population ratio by race and sex..	Bureau of Labor Statistics, Geographic Profile Series (stats.bls.gov/opub/gp/laugp htm). From this Web site page, select Estimates for Metropolitan Areas and Cities; tables available in PDF.
C. Distance traveled to work	
1. Share of metro employment >10 miles from central business district	Brookings Institution (www.brook.edu/es/urban/ publications/glaeserjobsprawlexsum.htm). Glaeser E.L., M. Kahn, and C. Chu 2001. Job Sprawl: Employment Location in U.S. Metropolitan Areas. Downloadable PDF.
D. Transportation system	
1. Percent of workers aged ≥16 years using various means of transportation to work	Census Bureau (www.census.gov).
2. Percent of residents without satisfactory public transportation available in neighborhood................................	American Housing Survey (www.census.gov/hhes/www/ahs.html). Data for each of 47 selected Metropolitan Areas are collected about every 4 years, with an average of 12 areas included each year. Downloadable data in SAS and ASCII formats.
5. Occupational Safety	
A. Laws, regulations, and company-specific policies	
1. Directory of states with approved occupational safety and health plans.............	Occupational Safety and Health Administration (www.osha.gov/oshdir/states.html).
B. Enforcement/number of violations	
1. OSHA workplace inspections and penalties for violations..	Occupational Safety and Health Administration Workplace Safety Data (www.nicar.org/data/osha). Businesses classified by city; data since 1972 available for purchase.

Continued on next page

Employment Data Sets, Continued

Components and Indicators	Data Sources and Notes
6. Job Quality	
A. Compensation..	See Economic Dimension, Income, page 6.
B. Ratio of Chief Executive Officer to worker earnings	
1. Ratio of mean annual wages, chief executives to production workers.................	Can be calculated from 1999 Occupational Employment Statistics data (www.bls.gov/oes/oes_data htm).
7. Job Characteristics	
A. Unionized companies/size and power of unions	See Workforce Characteristics, Unionization, page 15.
B. Skills needed by employers	
1. Percent of total employment in various industries...	Bureau of Economic Analysis (www.bea.doc.gov/bea/regional/reis). Can be calculated from data in downloadable compressed comma-separated-value files.
C. Full vs. part-time employment	
1. Percent of workers who work part-time........	Census Bureau (www.census.gov).

Education

Overview

Researchers studying educational context and health have generally used the percent of the adult population not completing high school as an indicator, finding positive associations with all-cause mortality (Guest and Almgren and Hussey 1998; Bosma et al. 2001), homicide (Cubbin and LeClere and Smith 2000), motor vehicle deaths (Cubbin and LeClere and Smith 2000), coronary heart disease prevalence (Diez Roux et al. 1997), neural tube defects (Wasserman et al. 1998), smoking (Diez Roux et al. 1997), severe pediatric injury (Durkin et al. 1994), and elevated serum cholesterol (Diez Roux et al. 1997). High school noncompletion rate and median educational level have also been used in combination with other areal economic and employment measures to form aggregate socioeconomic scores that are correlated with adverse health outcomes (Diez Roux et al. 2001; Roberts 1997).

In these studies the contextual educational variable tends to be treated as a marker for a more generalized concept of community socioeconomic status and resources, rather than being considered in its own right. Our consultants suggested that a focused assessment of aspects of education that are likely to vary among communities is warranted. Multiple measures of the population's educational attainment and functioning are included in the recommended indicators. Moreover, the levels of funding, characteristics of school systems and curricula, and learning-related aspects of community life such as prevalence of television viewing and numbers of library books per capita, can provide insights into the priority placed on education and corresponding investment within an area, which itself may be related to health outcome.

Specific aspects of the curriculum also have implications for the health of children at school ages and throughout their lives. For instance, bullying and violence is a serious problem among children and adolescents (Nansel et al. 2001), and the presence of violence prevention programs has been found to be effective in decreasing physically aggressive behavior (Twemlow et al. 2001; Grossman et al. 1997). Similarly, obesity in children is approaching epidemic proportions and is related to adult obesity; levels of lipids, cholesterol, triglycerides, insulin, and blood pressure; and risk of coronary heart disease (Styne 2001). Incorporation of nutrition modification programs and optimal physical education curricula in schools can be effective in modifying these risks (Stone et al. 1998; Snyder et al. 1999).

Education Data Sets

This table describes the components and indicators of the education dimension. Five education components are identified:
1. Educational Attainment
2. Funding
3. Private Schools
4. School Characteristics
5. Community Climate
Within each component, several indicators are identified, and for each indicator at least one data set is listed.

Components and Indicators	Data Sources and Notes
1. Educational Attainment	
A. Graduation rates	
1. Educational attainment among persons aged ≥25 years	Census Bureau (www.census.gov).
2. Number of diploma recipients; number of other high school completers	National Center for Education Statistics Common Core of Data (CCD). Downloadable comma-separated-value and Excel data tables for MSAs, counties, districts, and schools can be created with a Build a Table tool (nces.ed.gov/ccd/bat). Source CCD data sets also downloadable in ASCII format (nces.ed.gov/ccd/ccddata.asp).
3. High school graduation rates	U.S. Department of Education, No Child Left Behind (www nochildleftbehind.gov/index html). Starting with the 2002-03 school year, school districts will publicly report graduation rates.
B. Dropout rates	
1. Percent of persons aged 16-19 years not enrolled, not high school graduates	Census Bureau (www.census.gov).
2. Dropout rates for grades 7-12 and 9-12	CCD Local Education Agency (School District) Universe Dropout Data (nces.ed.gov/ccd/drpagency.asp); downloadable in ASCII format.
3. High school dropout rates................................	U.S. Department of Education, No Child Left Behind (www nochildleftbehind.gov/index html). Starting with the 2002-03 school year, school districts will publicly report dropout rates.
C. Literacy rates	
1. Reading assessment results	U.S. Department of Education, No Child Left Behind (www nochildleftbehind.gov/index html). Starting with the 2002-03 school year, school districts will publicly report test results.

Continued on next page

Education Data Sets, Continued

Components and Indicators	Data Sources and Notes
1. Educational Attainment (continued)	
D. Test scores	
1. Reading, math, and science assessment results	U.S. Department of Education, No Child Left Behind (www nochildleftbehind.gov/index html). Starting with the 2002-03 school year, school districts will publicly report test results.
2. Average SAT scores..	The College Board (www.collegeboard.com) releases data to states/districts.
E. Rates of progression to post-secondary education	
1. Post-secondary enrollment	Census Bureau (www.census.gov).
2. Funding	
A. Teacher salaries	
1. Mean annual wage: preschool, elementary, middle school, and secondary teachers	Bureau of Labor Statistics (stat.bls.gov/oes/home htm). Downloadable Excel files.
B. Facilities	
1. Percent of schools with at least one inadequate building feature..	National Education Association (www.nea.org/lac/modern/modchart html). State-level data.
C. Teacher training/support	
1. Professional qualifications of teachers	U.S. Department of Education, No Child Left Behind (www nochildleftbehind.gov/index html). Starting with the 2002-03 school year, school districts will publicly report this information.
2. Percent of expenditures on instructional staff support	School District Data Book (www.census.gov/mp/www/rom/msrom6i html). Data on CD-ROM available for purchase.
D. Fiscal capacity of school district	
1. Expenditures per pupil......................................	School District Data Book (www.census.gov/mp/www/rom/msrom6i html).
2. Long-term debt outstanding	School District Data Book (www.census.gov/mp/www/rom/msrom6i html).
E. Proportion of funds by source	
1. Revenues by source for public schools	School District Data Book (www.census.gov/mp/www/rom/msrom6i html).
2. Local government expenditures on education....	Census of Governments (www.census.gov/govs/www).
3. Consumer expenditures on education................	See Economic Dimension, Cost of Living, page 8.

Continued on next page

Education Data Sets, Continued

Components and Indicators	Data Sources and Notes
3. Private Schools	
A. Number	
1. Number of private schools	National Private Schools Association Group (www.npsag.com/database.html). Commercially available database on CD-ROM or diskette.
B. Enrollment	
1. Percent of students not enrolled in public school...	School District Data Book (www.census.gov/mp/www/rom/msrom6i html).
2. Enrollment in private schools............................	National Private Schools Association Group (www.npsag.com/database.html).
4. School Characteristics	
A. Size of schools/classes	
1. Public school enrollment.................................	School District Data Book (www.census.gov/mp/www/rom/msrom6i html). National Center for Health Statistics Common Core of Data (CCD) (nces.ed.gov/ccd/ccddata.asp).
2. Mean number of students in primary, middle, and high school..	Characteristics of the 100 Largest Public Elementary and Secondary School Districts in the United States (nces.ed.gov/pubs2001/100_largest/index.asp).
B. Student/teacher ratios	
1. Pupils per teacher	CCD. Downloadable comma-separated-value and Excel data tables for MSAs, counties, districts, and schools can be created with a Build a Table tool (nces.ed.gov/ccd/bat).
C. Teacher turnover	
1. Rates of teacher turnover.................................	Schools and Staffing Survey and Teacher Followup Survey (www.nces.ed.gov).
D. Parental attitude/involvement in schools	
1. Percent of households with children aged 0-13 years reporting unsatisfactory public schools in their neighborhood...	American Housing Survey (www.census.gov/hhes/www/ahs html). Data for each of 47 selected Metropolitan Areas are collected about every 4 years, with an average of 12 areas included each year. Downloadable data in SAS and ASCII formats.

Continued on next page

Education Data Sets, Continued

Components and Indicators	Data Sources and Notes
4. School Characteristics (continued)	
E. School segregation	
1. Race/ethnicity	
a. Enrollment by race/ethnicity......................	National Center for Education Statistics Common Core of Data (CCD). Downloadable comma-separated-value and Excel data tables for MSAs, counties, districts, and schools can be created with a Build a Table tool (nces.ed.gov/ccd/bat).
b. Exposure of minority students to white students..	Frankenberg, E., C. Lee, and G. Orfield. 2003. A Multiracial Society with Segregated Schools: Are We Losing the Dream? (www.civilrightsproject. harvard.edu/research/ reseg03/reseg03_full.php).
2. Economic status	
a. Percent of students eligible for free lunch	Can be calculated from data in the School District Data Book (www.census.gov/mp/www/rom/msrom6i html).
F. Curriculum quality	
1. Physical education requirements	
a. Mandated requirements for physical education	School Health Policies and Programs Study (www.cdc.gov/nccdphp/dash/shpps/index.htm). Data available in ASCII, SAS, and SPSS formats.
2. Health education	
a. Health education coordinator in place; health education standards required; curriculum required for accident/injury prevention, alcohol/drug use prevention, consumer health, CPR, death and dying, dental and oral health, emotional and mental health, first aid, growth and development, HIV prevention, immunizations, personal hygiene, suicide prevention, sun safety or skin cancer prevention, tobacco use, and violence prevention..	School Health Policies and Programs Study (www.cdc.gov/nccdphp/dash/shpps/index.htm).
3. Nutrition education	
a. Nutrition and dietary behavior curriculum required..	School Health Policies and Programs Study (www.cdc.gov/nccdphp/dash/shpps/index.htm).
4. Sex education	
a. Required curricula for human sexuality, pregnancy prevention, and STD prevention	School Health Policies and Programs Study (www.cdc.gov/nccdphp/dash/shpps/index.htm).

Continued on next page

Education Data Sets, Continued

Components and Indicators	Data Sources and Notes
4. School Characteristics (continued)	
G. Preschool/Kindergarten/Early Intervention	
1. Nursery school, preschool enrollment...............	Census Bureau (www.census.gov).
H. School-based clinics	
1. Number of school-based health centers	Center for Health and Health Care in Schools (www.healthinschools.org/home.asp).
I. Physical environment of school/safety	
1. On school property: availability of drugs; percent of students threatened/injured with a weapon, involved in physical fights, or carrying a weapon; percent of students who do not feel safe on school property; percent of teachers victimized	National Education Goals Panel (www.negp.gov).
5. Community Climate	
A. Television viewing	
1. Hours per week of television viewing, by age	Nielson Media Research (www.nielsonmedia.com).
B. Radio stations	
1. Number of radio stations	Gale Directory of Publications and Broadcast Media (galenet.gale.com/a/acp/db/gdpbm).
C. Reading/reading to children	
1. Proportion of households receiving daily newspapers	SRDS Corporation (www.srds.com).
2. Number of local newspapers	Gale Directory of Publications and Broadcast Media (galenet.gale.com/a/acp/db/gdpbm).
D. Libraries	
1. Number of libraries; number of library books and serial volumes	Public Libraries Survey (nces.ed.gov/surveys/libraries).

Political

Overview

Aspects of community political participation have been found to be associated with population health status. Davey Smith and Dorling (1996), for example, showed that in England and Wales, mortality rates in electoral constituencies were negatively correlated with Conservative voting patterns and positively correlated with Labour voting. Area deprivation was also negatively associated with Conservative voting but positively associated with Labour voting. The authors concluded that in areas with better material circumstances and more optimal health, voters were more likely to support leadership that favors reducing public assistance programs. In the United States, Blakely and colleagues (2001) studied disparities among states in voting across socioeconomic status groups. Individuals living in states with the highest voting inequality were shown to have increased odds of fair or poor self-rated health relative to those in other states. They reasoned that disproportionate political participation by the more economically well-off skews subsequent policy-making towards their interests, a conclusion supported in the political science literature (Hill and Leighley 1992).

More broadly, political participation has been of recent interest as an indicator of embeddedness in the institutions of civil society. As such, it is considered to be a reflection of social capital within a community (Kawachi 1999). Social capital, measured in several different ways, has been associated with positive health outcomes (Subramanian and Kawachi and Kennedy 2001; Kawachi and Kennedy and Glass 1999a; Kawachi et al. 1997) (see the Psychosocial Dimension, page 51, for further discussion of the social capital concept).

Within the political contextual dimension, we include aspects of political participation such as voting and political party membership, as well as donations to parties and candidates, which are known to influence public policy (Ferguson 1995). Likewise the degree to which elected officials are representative of their areas in terms of gender and race/ethnicity may be an important factor in their responsiveness to constituents' needs (Whitby 1997; Bratton and Haynie 1999). The percent of the local budget devoted to public health investments can be considered an indication of the priority placed on health by the community as well as a measure of available fiscal resources. We also include the number and influence of various politically active community groups.

Political Data Sets

This table describes the components and indicators of the political dimension. Three political components are identified:
1. Civic Participation
2. Political Structure
3. Power Groups
Within each component, several indicators are identified, and for each indicator at least one data set is listed.

Components and Indicators	Data Sources and Notes
1. Civic Participation	
A. Voting	
1. Voting and registration rates	
a. Votes cast for president, by party	USA Counties (www.census.gov/statab/www/county html). Data available on CD-ROM; online data for single counties downloadable as text or comma-separated-value file.
b. Percent of persons registered to vote and voting by race/ethnicity	Census Bureau (www.census.gov/prod/3/98pubs/p20-504u.pdf). State data in PDF.
2. Ease of registration	
a. Voter registration by mail allowed; registration deadline prior to election	Moving and Relocation Sourcebook and Directory (www.omnigraphics.com). Hardcover book available for purchase.
3. Racial/ethnic representativeness of registered voters...	See voting and registration rates above.
B. Census participation	
1. Census response rates...	Census Bureau (www.census.gov).
C. Political party membership	See voting and registration rates above.
D. Donations to parties and candidates	
1. Donations to Republican and Democratic candidates, parties, and political action committees..	Center for Responsive Politics (www.opensecrets.org). Contributions for selected metropolitan areas, zip codes, and states.

Continued on next page

Political Data Sets, Continued

Components and Indicators	Data Sources and Notes
2. Political Structure	
A. Gender/racial/ethnic representation in elected office	
1. Women in governing body	Carpenter, A. 1996. Facts About the Cities. New York: HW Wilson.
2. Elected officials in local governments by sex, race, and state	Census of Governments (www.census.gov/govs/www). From this Web site page, select Census of Governments for 1992; select Vol. 1, No. 2, Popularly Elected Officials. Available in PDF.
3. Percent of women in statewide elective office	Center for American Women and Politics (www.rci.rutgers.edu/~cawp).
4. Blacks in elected office......................................	Joint Center for Political and Economic Studies DataBank (www.jointcenter.org/DB/index htm).
B. Percent of local budget for public health investments	
1. Expenditures for health and welfare...................	Census of Governments (www.census.gov/govs/www). From this Web site page, select year of interest; select Vol. 4, No. 3, Finances of County Governments, or No. 4, Finances of Municipal and Township Governments. Downloadable spreadsheet or comma-separated-value files available.
3. Power Groups	
A. Community organizations	
1. Number and size of organizations: religious, political, civic and social, social advocacy, human rights, environmental and wildlife, business, labor, grant making and giving.	County Business Patterns (www.census.gov/epcd/cbp/view/cbp/view/cbpview.html). From this Web site page, select County, State, U.S., ZIP or MSA Database on a NAICS Basis. Select area of interest; in Number of Establishments table select detail for Industry Code 81, Other Services. Data downloadable as text or comma-separated-value tables; CD-ROM also available.
B. Unions..	See Employment Dimension, Workforce Characteristics, page 15.

Environmental

Overview

The environmental dimension includes physical and chemical components that have known associations with adverse health outcomes—air pollutants (American Lung Association 2001; Pope and Bates and Raizenne 1995); water pollutants (Griffith et al. 1989); and environmental hazards, including hazardous waste (Johnson 1999; Schell 1991), heavy metals (Goldman and Shannon and the American Academy of Pediatrics Committee on Environmental Health 2001; Mendelsohn et al. 1999), pesticides (Blindauer and Jackson and McGeehin 1999; Landrigan et al. 1999), climatic extremes (Greenough et al. 2001; Patz and McGeehin and Bernard 2001), and excessive noise (W. Passchier-Vermeer and W.F. Passchier 2000; Schell 1991). These exposures are known to vary by area and to be disproportionately concentrated among disadvantaged populations (American Lung Association 2001; Brown 1995).

In addition, this contextual dimension encompasses structural features of communities such as physical design of streets, sidewalks, and safety structures that are associated with level of injury risk (Navin and Zein and Felipe 2000; Agran et al. 1996). Aspects of land usage are also considered, such as public spaces and parks that may facilitate greater physical activity levels (French and Story and Jeffery 2001), as are services related to environmental quality like waste disposal and recycling programs.

Environmental Data Sets

This table describes the components and indicators of the environmental dimension. Five environmental components are identified:
1. Air Quality
2. Water Quality
3. Environmental Hazards
4. Physical Safety
5. Land Use

Within each component, several indicators are identified, and for each indicator at least one data set is listed.

Components and Indicators	Data Sources and Notes
1. Air Quality	
A. Outdoor	
1. Peak air concentration of carbon monoxide, lead, nitrogen dioxide, ozone, and sulfur dioxide; particulate matter air concentration; days Air Quality Index is higher than 100	Environmental Protection Agency (EPA) (www.epa.gov/airtrends). From this Web site page, select Metropolitan Area Trends; choose Table A-15 for Peak Concentrations or Table A-17 for Air Quality Index. Available in PDF.
2. Total pounds of air chemicals emitted by industry, by chemical	EPA, Toxics Release Inventory (www.epa.gov/tri). From this Web site page, select Get TRI Data; select TRI Explorer; under Chemical Released choose Select a Chemical Group, then Hazardous Air Pollutants; select geographic area of interest, then generate downloadable report.
B. Indoor	
1. Percent of households reporting neighborhood odor to be a problem or bothersome..................	American Housing Survey (www.census.gov/hhes/www/ahs.html). Data for each of 47 selected Metropolitan Areas are collected about every 4 years, with an average of 12 areas included each year. Downloadable data in SAS and ASCII formats.
2. Water Quality	
A. Number of violations per year for federally regulated drinking water contaminants...	EPA (www.epa.gov/safewater/data/pivottables.html#summdetails). Downloadable compressed Excel files.
B. Total pounds of surface water chemicals discharged by industry, by chemical	EPA, Toxics Release Inventory (www.epa.gov/tri). From this Web site page, select Get TRI Data; select TRI Explorer; select report by industry or chemical, choose geographic area of interest, then generate downloadable report.

Continued on next page

Environmental Data Sets, Continued

Components and Indicators	Data Sources and Notes
3. Environmental Hazards	
A. Hazardous waste	
1. Total pounds of chemical waste released by industry, by chemical	EPA, Toxics Release Inventory (www.epa.gov/tri). From this Web site page, select Get TRI Data; select TRI Explorer; select report by industry or chemical, choose geographic area of interest, then generate downloadable report.
B. Heavy metals	
1. Total pounds of selected heavy metals released by industry	EPA, Toxics Release Inventory (www.epa.gov/tri). From this Web site page, select Get TRI Data; select TRI Explorer; under Chemical Released choose Select a Chemical Group, then Metals and Metal Compounds; select geographic area of interest, then generate downloadable report.
C. Pesticides	
1. Total pounds of pesticide chemicals	EPA, Toxics Release Inventory (www.epa.gov/tri). From this Web site page, select Get TRI Data; select TRI Explorer; select report by industry or chemical, choose geographic area of interest, then generate downloadable report.
D. Climate extremes	
1. Maximum and minimum temperatures	Statistical Abstract of the United States (www.census.gov/statab/www). From this Web site page, select desired year, then Geography and Environment.
E. Noise	
1. Percent of households reporting noise to be a problem or bothersome	American Housing Survey (www.census.gov/hhes/www/ahs.html). Data for each of 47 selected Metropolitan Areas are collected about every 4 years, with an average of 12 areas included each year. Downloadable data in SAS and ASCII formats.
4. Physical Safety	
A. Traffic	
1. Total miles of local roads; total vehicle miles of local road travel daily	Federal Highway Administration (www.fhwa.dot.gov/policy/ohpi/hss/hsspubs htm). From this Web site page, select Highway Statistics for desired year; select Roadway Extent, Characteristics, and Performance. Available in PDF and Excel.
2. Percent of households perceiving traffic as a problem or bothersome	American Housing Survey (www.census.gov/hhes/www/ahs.html). Data for each of 47 selected Metropolitan Areas are collected about every 4 years, with an average of 12 areas included each year. Downloadable data in SAS and ASCII formats.

Continued on next page

Environmental Data Sets, Continued

Components and Indicators	Data Sources and Notes
4. Physical Safety (continued)	
B. Street repair	
1. Percent of households reporting major street repair needed in their neighborhood..................	American Housing Survey (www.census.gov/hhes/www/ahs.html). Data for each of 47 selected Metropolitan Areas are collected about every 4 years, with an average of 12 areas included each year. Downloadable data in SAS and ASCII formats.
5. Land Use	
A. Public recreational space/number of parks	
1 Expenditures on natural resources, parks, and recreation	Census of Governments (www.census.gov/govs/www). From this Web site page, select year of interest; select Vol. 4, No. 3, Finances of County Governments, or No. 4, Finances of Municipal and Township Governments, or select downloadable State and Local Government Finance data.
B. Waste disposal/dumping/sanitation services	
1. Pounds of waste managed	EPA, Toxics Release Inventory (www.epa.gov/tri). From this Web site page, select Get TRI Data; select TRI Explorer; select report by industry or chemical, then choose geographic area of interest; then choose waste quantity reports; generate downloadable report.
2. Percent of households reporting major trash, litter, or junk on streets near their home; reporting neighborhood litter/deterioration to be a problem or bothersome; and reporting poor city or county services in neighborhood	American Housing Survey (www.census.gov/hhes/www/ahs.html).
C. Curbside recycling programs	
1. Pounds of waste transferred to recycling	EPA, Toxics Release Inventory (www.epa.gov/tri). From this Web site page, select Get TRI Data; select TRI Explorer; select report by industry or chemical, then choose geographic area of interest; then choose waste quantity reports; generate downloadable report.

Housing

Overview

Associations between housing and health have been studied from several perspectives. Most concretely, physical characteristics of housing have been linked to adverse outcomes. For example, the presence of dampness and mold leads to increased risk of respiratory and other illnesses (Platt et al. 1989; Packer and Stewart-Brown and Fowle 1994). Dilapidated and abandoned housing in the local area increases the risk of accidental injury among residents (Gielen et al. 1995), is associated with increased emotional stress (Ellaway and Macintyre 2000), and may provide situational opportunities for high-risk behaviors (Cohen et al. 2000). Population density and overcrowding have also been associated with increased chances of contracting infections and sustaining injury (Agran et al. 1996; Acevedo-Garcia 2000).

Home ownership has been associated with reduced morbidity and mortality risk (Filakti and Fox 1995; O'Campo et al. 1997). In most cases this housing variable is regarded as a marker for general material well-being. It has been suggested, however, that long-term exposure to specific health promoting or damaging characteristics of housing itself is likely to account for some of the observed health effects (Macintyre et al. 1998; Ellaway and Macintyre 1998).

There is also some evidence that poor housing conditions during childhood can adversely affect health in later life. For example, Barker and colleagues (1990) found an association between domestic crowding during childhood and later stomach cancer mortality rates, suggesting that overcrowding may promote the transmission of causative organisms among children that exert negative health effects later in life. Similarly, Dedman et al. (2001) noted aspects of poorer childhood housing conditions were associated with increased mortality risk from common diseases in adulthood.

Our consultants suggested that we include these characteristics of housing in our framework, as well as other aspects of residential patterns within communities. Homelessness, for example, has known associations with differentially poorer health (Barrow et al. 1999; Hwang 2001). Segregation by race has been associated with adverse health outcomes among blacks (Williams and Collins 2001; Jackson et al. 2000), as well as among whites in some cases (Collins and Williams 1999). Similarly, concentration of poverty has been found to be associated with elevated mortality risk (Waitzman and Smith 1998a).

Continued on next page

31

We also include two other components within the housing dimension. Regulations such as zoning and industrial/residential segregation can affect the degree to which residential areas are exposed to industrial pollution and other health threats such as increased traffic. Financial issues specific to housing, such as housing costs, the availability and characteristics of low-income housing, mortgage lending practices, and community reinvestment initiatives are also considered.

Housing Data Sets

This table describes the components and indicators of the housing dimension. Four housing components are identified:
1. Housing Stock
2. Residential Patterns
3. Regulation
4. Financial Issues

Within each component, several indicators are identified, and for each indicator at least one data set is listed.

Components and Indicators	Data Sources and Notes
1. Housing Stock	
A. Age	
1. Median age of housing units	Census Bureau (www.census.gov).
2. New private housing units authorized by building permits as a percent of housing stock	1. State and Metropolitan Area Data Book (www.census.gov/statab/www/smadb html).
	2. State of the Nation's Housing (www.jchs.harvard.edu). From Web site page, choose publications, then most recent edition.
B. Scarcity	
1. Percent of housing units vacant.........................	Census Bureau (www.census.gov).
C. Value	
1. Median value, owner-occupied housing units....	Census Bureau (www.census.gov).
2. Median sales price of existing homes................	State of the Nation's Housing (www.jchs.harvard.edu). From Web site page, choose publications, then most recent edition.
4. Valuation of residential construction	See Economic Dimension, Fiscal Capacity, page 10.
D. Characteristics	
1. Percent of housing units lacking complete kitchen facilities, complete plumbing facilities, and/or telephone	Census Bureau (www.census.gov).
	American Housing Survey (www.census.gov/hhes/www/ahs.html). Data for each of 47 selected Metropolitan Areas are collected about every 4 years, with an average of 12 areas included each year. Downloadable data in SAS and ASCII formats.
2. Percent of households reporting 1 or more vandalized buildings in neighborhood; percent of households with best/worst opinion of their neighborhood (10 point scale)...........................	
E. Gentrification/gatedness	
1. Percent of home loans to high-income borrowers made in low-income areas of central cities..	State of the Nation's Housing (www.jchs.harvard.edu). From Web site page, choose publications, then most recent edition.
F. Rental vs. owner occupied	
1. Percent of occupied housing units that are owner occupied..	Census Bureau (www.census.gov).

Continued on next page

33

Housing Data Sets, Continued

Components and Indicators	Data Sources and Notes
2. Residential Patterns	
A. Homelessness	
1. Estimated homeless population	U.S. Conference of Mayors (usmayors.org/uscm/home.asp). From this Web site page, select Hunger and Homelessness from Reports and Publications.
B. Number of institutional facilities	
1. Number of homeless shelter beds; number of months wait for public housing and Section 8 vouchers	U.S. Conference of Mayors (usmayors.org/uscm/home.asp).
C. Segregation	
1. Racial/ethnic	
a. Indices of Dissimilarity, Isolation, Delta, Absolute Centralization, and Spatial Proximity	Iceland J., D. H. Weinberg, and E. Steinmetz. Racial and Ethnic Residential Segregation in the United States: 1980-2000. Census 2000 Special Report (landview.census.gov/hhes/www/housing/resseg/pdftoc html).
2. Economic	See Economic Dimension, Income, page 6.
D. Vacancy rates	
1. Percent of housing units vacant	Census Bureau (www.census.gov).
E. Crowded housing	
1. Mean number of persons per room	Census Bureau (www.census.gov).
F. Population density	
1. Persons per square mile	Census Bureau (www.census.gov).
3. Regulation	
A. Zoning policies	
1. Percent of households perceiving undesirable commercial, institutional, or industrial use as a problem or bothersome	American Housing Survey (www.census.gov/hhes/www/ahs.html). Data for each of 47 selected Metropolitan Areas are collected about every 4 years, with an average of 12 areas included each year. Downloadable data in SAS and ASCII formats.
B. Industrial/residential segregation	
1. Segregation indices for blacks, whites and Hispanics from high employment and hazardous manufacturing industries	Anderton D. L., and K. L. Egan. Industrial and Residential Segregation: Employment Opportunities and Environmental Burdens in Metropolitan Areas. (www.umass.edu/sadri/papers/wp20002.pdf).

Continued on next page

Housing Data Sets, Continued

Components and Indicators	Data Sources and Notes
4. Financial Issues	
A. Housing costs	
1. Cost of living index, housing and utilities; average 950 sq ft apartment rent, 2400 sq ft new home price, house payment, monthly energy costs	American Chamber of Commerce Researchers Association (www.accra.org). Quarterly and annual average data may be purchased as downloadable spreadsheet or hardcopy.
2. Basic family budgetary need for housing..........	Economic Policy Institute: Hardships in America (epinet.org). From this Web site page, choose Basic Family Budget Calculator; select a metropolitan area of interest or download budget tables for all areas in Excel.
3. Consumer expenditures on housing	Bureau of Labor Statistics (BLS) (www.bls.gov). From this Web site page, select Consumer Expenditures; select Tables Created by BLS; select current MSA tables grouped by region in text format or PDF.
4. Percent of income spent on mortgage/rent	American Housing Survey (www.census.gov/hhes/www/ahs.html). Data for each of 47 selected Metropolitan Areas are collected about every 4 years, with an average of 12 areas included each year. Downloadable data in SAS and ASCII formats.
5. Median gross rent as a percent of household income	Census Bureau (www.census.gov).
B. Low-income housing	
1. Percent of total housing	
a. Percentage of households receiving federal housing assistance	American Housing Survey (www.census.gov/hhes/www/ahs.html). Data for each of 47 selected Metropolitan Areas are collected about every 4 years, with an average of 12 areas included each year. Downloadable data in SAS and ASCII formats.
b. Percent of home loans to low-income borrowers..	State of the Nation's Housing (www.jchs.harvard.edu).
2. Ratio of low-income units to low-income workers.	
a. Ratio of low-rent units and Section 8 units to low-income families	Can be calculated from Housing Authority Profile data on low-rent units (www.hud.gov) and census data.
C. Mortgage lending practices by race/ethnicity	
1. Share of all home loans made to minority borrowers...	State of the Nation's Housing (www.jchs.harvard.edu).
2. Home loan denial rates by race	See Economy, Financial Services, page 8.
D. Community reinvestment initiatives	
1. Expenditures for housing and community development	Census of Governments (www.census.gov/govs/www). From this Web site page, select State and Local Government Finances; select year of interest. Downloadable spreadsheet or comma-separated-value files.

Medical

Overview

Health care services are generally considered to be an important determinant of health status (Andrulis 1998; Frenk 1998), although the degree to which medical care impacts health status over and above social and economic conditions has been the subject of considerable controversy (Pincus et al. 1998; McKeown 1979). The medical contextual dimension encompasses a range of health care services, including primary care, specialty care, emergency services, home health care, emergency services, mental health services, long-term care, oral health care, and alternative care.

We also look specifically at aspects of access to health care services, which is related to health status and known to vary among population groups (USDHHS 2000). Some of the factors included, such as insurance coverage and the availability of indigent care, are well-known determinants of access (Baker and Shapiro and Schur 2000; Newacheck et al. 1998; Nelson et al. 1999). The racial/ethnic makeup of medical staff in relation to the patient population and the cultural competence of providers and institutions may also be important in encouraging utilization of health care resources that are present in an area (Flores et al. 1998; Langer 1999). In addition to traditional measures of access, we also include rates of hospitalization for ambulatory care sensitive conditions. These are conditions considered to be manageable on an outpatient basis, given access to high-quality primary care, and therefore higher hospitalization rates can be used as an indicator of poorer access to appropriate care (Institute of Medicine 1993).

37

Medical Data Sets

This table describes the components and indicators of the medical dimension. Eight medical components are identified:

1. Primary Care
2. Specialty Care
3. Emergency Services
4. Home Health Care Services
5. Mental Health Care
6. Long-Term Care
7. Oral Health Care
8. Access to/Utilization of Care

Within each component, several indicators are identified, and for each indicator at least one data set is listed.

Components and Indicators	Data Sources and Notes
1. Primary Care	
A. Number of providers	
1. Total number of nonfederal MD/DOs in primary care, family practice, general practice, internal medicine, ob/gyn, and pediatric primary care practice................	American Medical Association Physicians Professional Data, Medical Marketing Service (www.mmslists.com/main.asp). Custom data tables in Excel may be purchased.
B. Provider training/competence/ certification	
1. Nonfederal physicians in primary care who are foreign medical graduates and who are board certified; hospital-associated medical staff who are board certified	Area Resource File (www.arfsys.com). Data available for purchase on CD-ROM, magnetic tape, and cartridge.
C. Medicaid/Medicare reimbursement levels	
1. Medicaid reimbursement rates for various medical services, including preventive care visits, immunization, critical care, emergency care, and surgery.....................................	American Academy of Pediatrics: Medicaid Reimbursement Survey (www.aap.org/research/medreimPDF01/all_states.PDF).
2. Age, sex, race, illness, and price-adjusted reimbursements for noncapitated Medicare per enrollee........	Dartmouth Atlas of Health Care (www.dartmouthatlas.org). Downloadable Excel files.

Continued on next page

Medical Data Sets, Continued

Components and Indicators	Data Sources and Notes
2. Specialty Care	
A. Number of providers	
1. Total number of nonfederal MD/DOs in medical and surgical specialty office practice	American Medical Association Physicians Professional data Medical Marketing Service (www.mmslists.com/main.asp). Custom data tables in Excel may be purchased.
B. Provider training/competence/ certification	
1. Nonfederal physicians in specialty care who are foreign medical graduates, and who are board certified; hospital-associated medical staff who are board certified	Area Resource File (www.arfsys.com).
3. Emergency Services	
A. Number of nonfederal physicians in emergency medicine patient care; number of hospitals with emergency departments	Area Resource File (www.arfsys.com).
4. Home Health Care Services	
A. Number of hospitals with home health services	Area Resource File (www.arfsys.com).
5. Mental Health Care	
A. Total number of nonfederal physicians in psychiatric, office-based patient care; number of hospitals with psychiatric emergency, outpatient, emergency social work, and outpatient social work services	Area Resource File (www.arfsys.com).
6. Long-Term Care	
A. Number of nursing and board-and-care homes and beds; number of long-term hospitals and beds	Area Resource File (www.arfsys.com).
7. Oral Health Care	
A. Total number of active dentists in private practice....................................	Area Resource File (www.arfsys.com).

Continued on next page

Medical Data Sets, Continued

Components and Indicators	Data Sources and Notes
8. Access to/Utilization of Care	
A. Insurance coverage	
1. Percent of persons aged 0-64 years who are uninsured, have job-based insurance, have no usual care source, and who delayed or went without needed care......	Brown, E. R., R. Wyn, and S. Teleki. 2000. Disparities in Health Insurance and Access to Care for Residents Across U.S. Cities. (www.cmwf.org/programs/insurance/ Brown85MSAsreport.pdf).
B. Race/ethnicity staff-to-population ratios	
1. Race/ethnicity staff-to-population ratios for primary care family practice, general practice, pediatric practice, internal medicine, ob/gyn, and medical and surgical subspecialties............................	Can be calculated from American Medical Association Physicians Professional Data, Medical Marketing Service (www mmslists.com) and census data.
C. Provision of care in total and indigent care	
1. Number of short-term general hospital admissions and emergency hospital outpatient visits	Area Resource File (www.arfsys.com).
D. Costs of care	
1. Average cost of routine MD visit, hospital room..	American Chamber of Commerce Researchers Association (www.accra.org). Quarterly and annual average data may be purchased as downloadable spreadsheet or hardcopy.
2. Consumer expenditures on health care	Bureau of Labor Statistics (BLS) (www.bls.gov). From this Web site page, select Consumer Expenditures; select Tables Created by BLS; select current MSA tables grouped by region in text format or PDF.
E. Rates of ambulatory care sensitive hospitalizations	
1. Rates of ambulatory care sensitive hospitalizations per 1,000 Medicare enrollees	Dartmouth Atlas of Health Care (www.dartmouthatlas.org).

Governmental

Overview

Within this dimension, we consider characteristics and functioning of local area governments. Levels of funding are assessed, as well as the relative contributions from various revenue sources. Policies and legislation that have potential health effects, such as obstacles to unionization and living wage or minimum wage ordinances and employer requirements for provision of health benefits, are included. The nature and quality of local governmental services are also considered.

Another aspect of local governance with potential health relevance concerns the degree to which there is municipal fragmentation. This term refers to a situation in which large numbers of smaller governmental entities exist within a metropolitan area. It has been argued that in cases where there are high levels of municipal fragmentation and no single government empowered to act for the good of the entire region, a host of problems result, including resource and public service imbalances within the area and the protection of privilege (Mitchell-Weaver and Miller and Deal 2000; Ross and Levine 1996).

Governmental Data Sets

This table describes the components and indicators of the governmental dimension. Four governmental components are identified.
1. Funding
2. Policy/Legislation
3. Services
4. Municipal Fragmentation (number of subunit governments within a metro area)

Within each component, several indicators are identified, and for each indicator at least one data set is listed.

Components and Indicators	Data Sources and Notes

1. Funding
 	
A. Revenue
 	
  1. Intergovernmental
    a. Revenue from federal, state, and local government sources...............
	Census of Governments (www.census.gov/govs/www). From this Web site page, select year of interest; select Vol. 4, No. 3, Finances of County Governments, or No. 4, Finances of Municipal and Township Governments. Downloadable spreadsheet or comma-separated-value files available.

2. Taxes a. Revenue from all taxes, property, income, and sales taxes	Census of Governments (www.census.gov/govs/www). From this Web site page, select State and Local Government Finances; select year of interest. Downloadable spreadsheet or comma-separated-value files.
3. Lottery a. Revenue from lottery............	Christiansen Capital Advisors (www.cca-i.com). From this Web site page, select Research; select Lottery Data. Excel files available for purchase.
B. Debt 1. Total debt outstanding................	Census of Governments (www.census.gov/govs/www). From this Web site page, select year of interest; select Vol. 4, No. 3, Finances of County Governments, or No. 4, Finances of Municipal and Township Governments. Downloadable spreadsheet or comma-separated-value files available.

Continued on next page

Governmental Data Sets, Continued

Components and Indicators	Data Sources and Notes
2. Policy/Legislation	
A. Obstacles to unionization	See Employment, Workforce Characteristics, page 15.
B. Living wage/minimum wage ordinances	
1. Living wage laws enacted	ACORN Living Wage Resource Center (www.acorn.org). From this Web site page, select Living Wage; select List of Cities and Counties Where Living Wage Ordinances Have Been Passed.
2. Minimum wage rate	U.S. Department of Labor (www.dol.gov/esa/minwage/america htm). Interactive map providing details of state minimum wage rates.
3. Services	
A. Privatization	
1. Number of state programs and services privatized..	Reason Public Policy Institute Privatization Center (www.privatization.org). From this Web site page, select Privatization Database; select Statistics and Trends. Results of surveys on number of programs and services privatized by state.
B. Local services/safety net resources	
1. Percent of households reporting poor levels of city or county services and reporting poor levels of police protection in their neighborhood	American Housing Survey (www.census.gov/hhes/www/ahs.html). Data for each of 47 selected Metropolitan Areas are collected about every 4 years, with an average of 12 areas included each year. Downloadable data in SAS and ASCII formats.
2. Expenditures on public welfare, health and hospitals, police and fire protection, parks and recreation, sewerage and sold waste management	Census of Governments (www.census.gov/govs/www). From this Web site page, select year of interest; select Vol. 4, No. 3, Finances of County Governments, or No. 4, Finances of Municipal and Township Governments. Downloadable spreadsheet or comma-separated-value files available.
4. Municipal fragmentation	
A. Number of local governments..............	Census of Governments (www.census.gov/govs/www). From this Web site page, select year of interest; select Vol. 1, No. 1, Government Organization, or downloadable spreadsheet or comma-separated-value files.
B. Metropolitan power diffusion index.....	Mitchell-Weaver, C., D. Miller, and R. Deal. 2000. Multilevel Governance and Metropolitan Regionalism in the U.S.A. Urban Studies 37(5-6):851-76.

Public Health

Overview

This dimension includes assessment of the implementation of core public health functions of assessment, policy development, and assurance at the local level (Turnlock and Handler 1997; Institute of Medicine 1988). We focus on three primary areas of interest. First, there are a variety of programs aimed at prevention, early detection, and optimal management of a range of health problems. Local public health departments may provide these services directly or oversee their implementation by other organizations, both governmental and private sector. The next category concerns development, regulation, and enforcement of standards, which has become a salient issue because provision of traditional public health services is increasingly being privatized (Beauchamp 1997). Thirdly, funding issues including budget allocations and financial arrangements for service provision are of interest in gauging the priority given to public health issues in the community.

Public Health Data Sets

This table describes the components and indicators of the public health dimension. Three public health components are identified:
1. Programs
2. Regulation/Enforcement
3. Funding
Within each component, several indicators are identified, and for each indicator at least one data set is listed.

Components and Indicators	Data Sources and Notes
1. Programs	
A. Screening..	
B. Nutrition...	
C. Family planning.................................	Local Health Department Infrastructure Study (www.sscnet.ucla.edu/issr/da/index/techinfo/i31851 htm). This survey addressed the paucity of current data on the U.S. public health infrastructure. Respondents' state identification only obtainable if user agrees to terms and conditions of a Restricted Data Use Agreement. Data available through the Inter-University Consortium for Political and Social Research; Stata file.
D. Chronic disease control.......................	
E. Home visiting	
F. Outreach..	
G. School-based clinics/education.............	
H. Substance abuse prevention................	
I. Domestic violence program	
J. Mental health services	
K. Immunization	
1. Percent of children aged 19-35 months completely immunized, by race/ethnicity	National Immunization Program (www.cdc.gov/nip/coverage/default.htm). From this Web site page, select National Immunization Survey (NIS); select NIS Data Tables; downloadable tables in Excel or HTML for states and select counties.
2. Regulation/Enforcement	
A. Sanitation	Local Health Department Infrastructure Study (www.sscnet.ucla.edu/issr/da/index/techinfo/i31851 htm).
B. Health/food inspection	
C. Health violations.................................	

Continued on next page

Public Health Data Sets, Continued

Components and Indicators	Data Sources and Notes
3. Funding	
A. Budget allocations	
1. Local health department expenditures.....	Local Health Department Infrastructure Study (www.sscnet.ucla.edu/issr/da/index/techinfo/i31851 htm).
2. Governmental expenditures on health.....	Census of Governments (www.census.gov/govs/www). From this Web site page, select year of interest; select Vol. 4, No. 3, Finances of County Governments, or No. 4, Finances of Municipal and Township Governments. Downloadable spreadsheet or comma-separated-value files available.
B. Private sector provision of public health services	
1. Percent of total local health department budget from private sources	Local Health Department Infrastructure Study (www.sscnet.ucla.edu/issr/da/index/techinfo/i31851 htm).

Psychosocial

Overview

There has been longstanding scientific interest in the organization of social life and the implications of interpersonal and group interactions for emotional and physical health status (House and Landis and Umberson 1988; Yen and Syme 1999). Research in the 1970s on social support suggested a health-enhancing role for social relationships in buffering the ill effects of stress (Cassel 1976), and subsequent studies confirmed an inverse relationship between social relationships and mortality risk (House and Robbins and Metzner 1982; Schoenbach et al. 1986).

More recently, aspects of social interactions and relationships have been increasingly conceptualized as forms of social capital, although there is widespread disagreement about the meaning of the term and the level of aggregation at which it operates (Lynch et al. 2000b; Woolcock 2001). Portes (1998) defines social capital as "the ability of actors to secure benefits by virtue of membership in social networks or other social structures." Coleman (1988) sees social capital as a resource for organizations as well as individuals: "Social capital is defined by its function. It is not a single entity but a variety of different entities, with two elements in common: they all consist of some aspect of social structures, and they facilitate certain actions of actors—whether persons or corporate actors—within the structure. Like other forms of capital, social capital is productive, making possible the achievement of certain ends that in its absence would not be possible." Putnam et al. (1993) considers social capital broadly as "features of social organization, such as trust, norms, and networks that can improve the efficiency of society by facilitating coordinated actions."

Social capital has been operationalized in different ways in health-related empirical research. Per capita membership in groups and associations has been used to assess civic engagement (Kawachi et al. 1997; Kawachi and Kennedy and Glass 1999a), as has political participation (Blakely and Kennedy and Kawachi 2001). Several studies have considered greater mistrust to be indicative of lower levels of social capital (Kawachi et al. 1997; Kawachi and Kennedy and Glass 1999a; Subramanian and Kawachi and Kennedy 2001). Mistrust is generally defined as the percent of persons in an area who agree with the second part of the following question: "Generally speaking, would you say that most people can be trusted or that you can't be too careful in dealing with people?"

Continued on next page

A related indicator is perceived lack of fairness, indexed by the percent of persons who agree that "most people would try to take advantage of you if they got the chance" (Kawachi et al. 1997). Perceived helpfulness/reciprocity has also been used as a gauge of social capital, based on answers to the question, "Would you say that most of the time people try to be helpful, or are they mostly looking out for themselves?" (Kawachi et al. 1997). It has also been hypothesized that crime level is an indicator of collective well-being that is influenced by the degree of cohesiveness in social relations or social capital (Sampson and Raudenbush and Earls 1997; Kawachi and Kennedy and Wilkinson 1999b).

Within the psychosocial dimension, we include theorized aspects of social capital such as civic engagement via political participation, membership in voluntary organizations and unions, and charitable giving. Crime as a marker for social cohesion is assessed through expenditures on jails and incarceration rates. Collection of information on lawsuits and the presence and utilization of protective services was also suggested as an indicator of the level of trust in communities.

Psychosocial Data Sets

This table describes the components and indicators of the psychosocial dimension. Seven psychosocial components are identified:
1. Political
2. Volunteer Organizations
3. Union Participation
4. Charitable Giving
5. Jails
6. Lawsuits
7. Protective Services

Within each component, several indicators are identified, and for each indicator at least one data set is listed.

Components and Indicators	Data Sources and Notes
1. Political	
A. Contributions to parties, candidates	See Political Dimension, Civic Participation, page 26.
B. Women in elected office	See Political Dimension, Political Structure, page 27.
C. Registered voters	See Political Dimension, Civic Participation, page 26.
2. Volunteer Organizations	
A. Types/functions	
1. Number of churches, total and by denomination	*Religious Congregations and Membership in the United States: 2000* (www.glenmary.org/grc/default.htm). Regional, state, and county data based on reporting from 149 religious bodies. Available for purchase as CD-ROM and hardcopy.
B. Number of members	
1. Number of church members and church adherents, total and by denomination	*Religious Congregations and Membership in the United States: 2000* (www.glenmary.org/grc/default.htm).
2. Number and size of membership organizations, including churches and political and civic organizations	See Political Dimension, Power Groups, page 27.
3. Union Participation	See Employment Dimension, Workforce Characteristics, page 15.
4. Charitable Giving	
1. Average charitable contribution per itemized income tax return; number of public charitable organizations by type of charity; monetary public support for public charitable organizations by type of charity	National Center for Charitable Statistics (nccsdataweb.urban.org/NCCS/Public). Data from the Internal Revenue Service and other sources; dataweb in development that will allow data viewing, extraction, and downloading.

Continued on next page

Psychosocial Data Sets, Continued

Components and Indicators	Data Sources and Notes
5. Jails	
A. Expenditures	
1. State and local justice system expenditures..	Sourcebook of Criminal Justice Statistics (www.albany.edu/ sourcebook). Data available online and in CD-ROM and print format.
2. Corrections expenditures.........................	Census of Governments (www.census.gov/govs/www). From this Web site page, select year of interest; select Vol. 4, No. 3, Finances of County Governments, or No. 4, Finances of Municipal and Township Governments. Downloadable spreadsheet or comma-separated-value files available.
B. Incarceration rates	
1. Average daily population in local jails; state prison incarceration rates	Bureau of Justice Statistics, Prison and Jail Inmates at Midyear (www.ojp.usdoj.gov/bjs/pubalp2 htm). PDF, ASCII, and spreadsheet files available for download.
2. Confined jail inmates by race, as a percent of total race specific population	Can be calculated from Bureau of Justice Statistics and census data.
C. Crime	
1. Number of serious crimes known to police	U.S. Counties (www.census.gov/statab/www/county html). Data available on CD-ROM; online data for single counties downloadable as text or comma-separated-value file.
6. Lawsuits	
A. Civil lawsuits	
1. Number of tort trials	Bureau of Justice Statistics: Tort Trials and Verdicts in Large Counties (www.ojp.usdoj.gov/bjs/pubalp2.htm). PDF, ASCII, and spreadsheet files available for download.
7. Protective Services	
A. Government services	
1. Police protection expenditures	Census of Governments (www.census.gov/govs/www). From this Web site page, select year of interest; select Vol. 4, No. 3, Finances of County Governments, or No. 4, Finances of Municipal and Township Governments. Downloadable spreadsheet or comma-separated-value files available.
2. Percent of households reporting poor levels of police protection in their neighborhood..	American Housing Survey (www.census.gov/hhes/www/ahs html). Data for each of 47 selected Metropolitan Areas are collected about every 4 years, with an average of 12 areas included each year. Downloadable data in SAS and ASCII formats.

Behavioral

Overview

As mentioned earlier, there has been increasing recognition that aspects of social, physical, and cultural context can affect health status in a community by facilitating or inhibiting behaviors that impact well-being (Macintyre and Ellaway and Cummins 2002). We focus on behavior areas that are among the nation's leading health indicators and that have been repeatedly cited as major determinants of premature morbidity and mortality—tobacco use, physical activity, diet/obesity, alcohol and illicit drug use, and violence (USDHHS 2000; McGinnis and Foege 1998; Wilson 1994).

For each of these behaviors, we examine specific characteristics of communities that might influence the degree to which they will be adopted by residents. In the case of tobacco use, these characteristics include current smoking rates, the presence of cessation and preventive education programs, workplace smoking restrictions, the cost and accessibility of cigarettes, and targeted advertising. In the area of physical activity, we include reported activity levels, physical education requirements in schools, participation in local sports and recreational activities, as well as availability of exercise facilities in the workplace and in the area more generally. We also consider indicators of sedentary activities such as television viewing patterns and video game sales and use. Regarding diet and obesity, we look at consumption patterns of healthy foods such as fruit and vegetables as well as high-fat and high-sugar foods. The quality, availability, and cost of a range of different foods is of interest, as is the availability of generally less nutritious "fast food" as indexed by the number of such establishments in the area. We also include aspects of nutrition in the schools, including the prevalence of subcontracting to vendors of non-nutritious items and the presence of nutrition education programs. In the area of alcohol and illicit drug use, we consider availability as indicated by the number of liquor stores, as well as marketing laws and the nature of public advertising. We also include drug and alcohol treatment service availability and the presence of syringe laws and exchange programs. Violence in the community is indicated by factors such as the availability of guns and the level of exposure to violence perceived by residents.

Behavioral Data Sets

This table describes the components and indicators of the behavioral dimension. Five behavioral components are identified:
1. Tobacco Use
2. Physical Activity
3. Diet/Obesity
4. Alcohol and Illicit Drug Use
5. Violence

Within each component, several indicators are identified, and for each indicator at least one data set is listed.

Components and Indicators	Data Sources and Notes
1. Tobacco Use	
A. Smoking rates	
1. Rate of ever smoking; number of cigarettes smoked per day; current smoking rates among adults	Behavioral Risk Factor Surveillance System (www.cdc.gov/brfss). Data for states available in Rich Text Format and SAS format. Estimates for Metropolitan Areas are available in the SMART BRFSS.
2. Current smoking rates among children in grades 6-8 and 9-12	National Tobacco Control Program State Exchange (www.cdc.gov/tobacco/ntcp_exchange/index.htm). This Web site page has links to state information.
B. Cessation programs	
1. Directory of local smoking cessation programs	Quitnet National Directory (www.quitnet.com/library/programs).
C. Smoking prevention	
1. Tobacco control funding	National Tobacco Control Program State Exchange (www.cdc.gov/tobacco/ntcp_exchange/index.htm).
D. Workplace/public space smoking restriction laws	
1. Workplace smoking policies	Behavioral Risk Factor Surveillance System (www.cdc.gov/brfss).
2. Smoking restrictions: government and private workplaces, restaurants, child day care, bars, malls, grocery stores, enclosed arenas, public transportation, hospitals, prisons, hotels, and motels	National Tobacco Control Program State Exchange (www.cdc.gov/tobacco/ntcp_exchange/index.htm).
E. Cost/accessibility of cigarettes	
1. Cigarette tax..	See Economic Dimension, Redistribution (Taxes), page 9.
2. Average local price of cigarettes	See Economic Dimension, Cost of Living, page 8.

Continued on next page

Behavioral Data Sets, Continued

Components and Indicators	Data Sources and Notes
2. Physical Activity	
A. Physical activity levels	
1. Type, frequency, and duration of physical activity.................................	Behavioral Risk Factor Surveillance System (www.cdc.gov/brfss).
B. Physical education requirements in schools...	See Education Dimension, School Characteristics, page 22.
C. Public and private recreational facilities	
1. Expenditures on natural resources, parks, and recreation...............................	Census of Governments (www.census.gov/govs/www). From this Web site page, select year of interest; select Vol. 4, No. 3, Finances of County Governments, or No. 4, Finances of Municipal and Township Governments. Downloadable spreadsheet or comma-separated-value files available.
D. Television viewing patterns	See Education Dimension, Community Climate, page 24.
3. Diet/Obesity	
A. Fresh fruit and vegetable consumption	
1. Food intake history	Behavioral Risk Factor Surveillance System (www.cdc.gov/brfss).
B. High-fat, high-sugar food consumption	
1. Food intake history	Behavioral Risk Factor Surveillance System (www.cdc.gov/brfss).
C. Food quality/availability	
1. Number of supermarkets, convenience stores..	Economic Census (www.census.gov). Data for specific types of retail trade companies available online and on CD-ROM.
2. Percent of food sales that are supermarket sales...................................	Progressive Grocers Market Scope (www.progressivegrocer.com).
3. Percent of households reporting unsatisfactory shopping in their neighborhood...............................	American Housing Survey (www.census.gov/hhes/www/ahs html). Data for each of 47 selected Metropolitan Areas are collected about every 4 years, with an average of 12 areas included each year. Downloadable data in SAS and ASCII format.
D. Number of fast food establishments	
1. Number of fast food restaurants...............	Economic Census (www.census.gov).
E. School nutrition	
1. Regulation of subcontracting to vendors	Commercial Activities in Schools GAO Report (www.gao.gov/archive/2000/he00156.pdf).
2. Nutrition education................................	See Education Dimension, School Characteristics, page 22.

Continued on next page

Behavioral Data Sets, Continued

Components and Indicators	Data Sources and Notes
4. Alcohol and Illicit Drug Use	
A. Number of beer, wine, and liquor stores	Economic Census (www.census.gov).
B. Drug and alcohol treatment services	
1. Number of hospitals with outpatient alcohol/drug abuse services; number of alcohol/chemical dependency treatment beds..	Area Resource File (www.arfsys.com). Data available for purchase on CD-ROM, magnetic tape, and cartridge.
2. Number of alcohol/chemical dependency treatment programs................................	Substance Abuse and Mental Health Services Administration facility locator (findtreatment.samhsa.gov/ facilitylocatordoc htm).
C. Syringe laws/exchange programs	
1. Law allowing sterile syringe exchange ...	Hard Truth About AIDS: Sterile Syringe Exchange Programs (hardtruth.qti.net/sterile_syringe_exchange_program.htm).
5. Violence	
A. Guns	
1. Availability	
a. Presence of firearms in home/vehicle	Behavioral Risk Factor Surveillance System (www.cdc.gov/brfss).
b. Number of gun stores	Economic Census (www.census.gov).
B. Exposure to violence	
1. Rates of violent crime.............................	FBI Uniform Crime Reports (www.fbi.gov/ucr/ucr htm). From this Web site page, select Crime in the United States; select year of interest; select Index of Crime for MSAs; data downloadable in Excel and PDF.
2. Perception of neighborhood safety	Behavioral Risk Factor Surveillance System (www.cdc.gov/brfss).
3. Percent of households perceiving neighborhood crime as a problem or bothersome	American Housing Survey (www.census.gov/hhes/www/ahs html). Data for each of 47 selected Metropolitan Areas are collected about every 4 years, with an average of 12 areas included each year. Downloadable data in SAS and ASCII formats.
C. Police protection.................................	See Psychosocial Dimension, Protective Services, page 54.

Transport

Overview

The transportation system in place in communities has multiple implications for the health of residents. Most directly, motor vehicles are the leading cause of injury in the United States and are responsible for about one-third of all injury deaths (Fingerhut and Warner 1997). The nature of the transportation modes and the volume of use also influence the types and magnitude of pollution introduced into the environment (Sharpe 1999). A third consideration is the degree to which employment patterns and therefore economic well-being are determined by the accessibility of jobs through adequate and affordable transportation systems (Pugh 1998).

In our framework we include measures within each of these health-related aspects of transportation. Vehicle occupant and pedestrian safety factors are included, as well as characteristics of the infrastructure of roads, sidewalks, and bike lanes. We examine characteristics and numbers of vehicles and aspects of the public transportation system. Finally, we include economic issues such as government transportation spending priorities, funding for public transportation, and personal insurance rates.

Transport Data Sets

This table describes the components and indicators of the transport dimension. Six transport components are identified:
1. Safety
2. Infrastructure
3. Traffic Patterns
4. Vehicles
5. Public Transportation
6. Economic Issues

Within each component, several indicators are identified, and for each indicator at least one data set is listed.

Components and Indicators	Data Sources and Notes
1. Safety	
A. Seat belts/child restraints	
1. Prevalence of seat belt and child safety seat use	Behavioral Risk Factor Surveillance System (www.cdc.gov/brfss). Data for states available in Rich Text Format and SAS; estimates for Metropolitan Areas under development by CDC.
B. Helmets	
1. Prevalence of child bicycle helmet use	Behavioral Risk Factor Surveillance System (www.cdc.gov/brfss).
C. Age curfews/graduated driver's license program	
1. Driver's license requirements for young drivers	Insurance Institute for Highway Safety/Highway Loss Data Institute (www hwysafety.org/). From this Web site page, select How States Measure Up.
D. Driving while intoxicated laws/enforcement	
1. Rating of driving while intoxicated laws and law enforcement	MADD (www.madd.org/home). From this Web site page, select Stats and Resources; select Laws; select Rating the States.
E. Speed restriction/enforcement	
1. Speed limit on urban interstates	Insurance Institute for Highway Safety/Highway Loss Data Institute (www hwysafety.org). From this Web site page, select How States Measure Up.
2. Peak period freeway and principal artery speed	Texas Transportation Institute (mobility.tamu.edu). Annual Urban Mobility Report includes speed and congestion information.

Continued on next page

Transport Data Sets, Continued

Components and Indicators	Data Sources and Notes

2. Infrastructure
 	
A. Roads
 	
  1. Quantity
    a. Miles of interstate, other freeways, and expressways; other principal arteries, minor arterial, collector, and local roads; total roadway miles ....
	Federal Highway Administration (www.fhwa.dot.gov/policy/ohpi/hss/hsspubs.htm). From this Web site page, select Highway Statistics for desired year; select Roadway Extent, Characteristics, and Performance. PDF and Excel files.

2. Quality a. Percent of households reporting major repairs needed to streets in their neighborhood...........................	American Housing Survey (www.census.gov/hhes/www/ahs html). Data for each of 47 selected Metropolitan Areas are collected about every 4 years, with an average of 12 areas included each year. Downloadable data in SAS and ASCII formats.
3. Traffic Patterns **A. Spatial location of jobs** 1. Mean travel time to work, workers aged $\geq$16 years; average daily commute distance	Census Bureau (www.census.gov).
B. Traffic volume 1. Vehicle miles of local road traveled daily, total and by type of road; travel time index (measure of congestion at peak times); percent of lane miles with congestion...............................	Texas Transportation Institute (mobility.tamu.edu).
2. Percent of households reporting street noise or traffic as a problem or bothersome	American Housing Survey (www.census.gov/hhes/www/ahs html). Data for each of 47 selected Metropolitan Areas are collected about every 4 years, with an average of 12 areas included each year. Downloadable data in SAS and ASCII formats.
3. Annual traffic growth rates	Highway and Motorway Fact Book (www.publicpurpose.com/ut-ushyg htm).
C. Car pooling 1. Percent of workers aged $\geq$16 years carpooling to work.................................	Census Bureau (www.census.gov).

Continued on next page

Transport Data Sets, Continued

Components and Indicators	Data Sources and Notes
4. Vehicles	
A. Numbers of vehicles	
1. Vehicles available per household.............	Census Bureau (www.census.gov).
B. Types of vehicles	
1. Numbers of automobiles, buses, trucks, and trailers registered	Federal Highway Administration (www.fhwa.dot.gov/policy/ohpi/hss/hsspubs.htm). From this Web site page, select Highway Statistics for desired year; select Motor Vehicles. PDF and Excel files.
5. Public Transportation	
A. Availability/density/efficiency	
1. Percent of households reporting unsatisfactory or no public transportation in their neighborhood.......	American Housing Survey (www.census.gov/hhes/www/ahs html). Data for each of 47 selected Metropolitan Areas are collected about every 4 years, with an average of 12 areas included each year. Downloadable data in SAS and ASCII formats.
B. Types of public transportation available	
1. Percent of workers aged $\geq$16 years using various means of transportation to work	Census Bureau (www.census.gov).
C. Cohesiveness/integration	
1. Percent of trips taken by car, by transit, on foot, and by bicycle	Driven to Spend: The Impact of Sprawl on Household. Expenses (www.transact.org). From this Web site page, select Library; select STPP Reports.
6. Economic Issues	
A. Expenditures	
1. Highway expenditures............................	Census of Governments (www.census.gov/govs/www). From this Web site page, select year of interest; select Vol. 4, No. 3, Finances of County Governments, or No. 4, Finances of Municipal and Township Governments, or downloadable State and Local Government Finance data.
2. Percent of total household expenditures for transportation; household spending on public transportation..........................	Driven to Spend: The Impact of Sprawl on Household Expenses (www.transact.org).
3. Consumer expenditures on transportation...	See Economic Dimension, Cost of Living, page 9.

Continued on next page

Transport Data Sets, Continued

Components and Indicators	Data Sources and Notes
6. Economic Issues (continued)	
B. Spending on local roads vs. alternative transportation	
1. Funding for state grants-in-aid for mass transit; funding for highway	Federal Highway Administration (www.fhwa.dot.gov/policy/ohpi/hss/hsspubs.htm). From this Web site page, select Highway Statistics for desired year; select Highway Finance. PDF and Excel files.
C. Percent of transit revenue from fares	
1. Percent of total operating funds that are fare revenues..	National Transit Database (www.fta.dot.gov/ntl/database.html). PDF and HTML tables.
D. Insurance rates	
1. Average expenditure for auto insurance	See Economic Dimension, Cost of Living, page 9.
E. Commuter taxes	
1. Transit and vanpool tax exemption benefits	See Economic Dimension, Exploitation (Commuter Taxes), page 11.

References

This chapter lists references for the text.

Acevedo-Garcia, D. 2000. "Residential Segregation and the Epidemiology of Infectious Diseases." Social Science and Medicine 51:1143-61.

Agran, P. F., D. G. Winn, C. L. Anderson, C. Tran, and C. P. Del Valle. 1996. "The Role of the Physical and Traffic Environment in Child Pedestrian Injuries." Pediatrics 98(6 pt 2):1096-103.

American Lung Association. 2001. "Urban Air Pollution and Health Inequalities: A Workshop Report." Environmental Health Perspectives 109(suppl 3):357-74.

Anderson, R. T., P. Sorlie, E. Backlund, N. Johnson, and G. A. Kaplan. 1997. "Mortality Effects of Community Socioeconomic Status." Epidemiology 8:42-7.

Andrulis, D. P. 1998. "Access to Care is the Centerpiece in the Elimination of Socioeconomic Disparities in Health." Annals of Internal Medicine 129:412-6.

Armstrong, D. L., E. Barnett, M. Casper, and S. Wing. 1998. "Community Occupational Structure, Medical and Economic Resources, and Coronary Mortality among U.S. Blacks and Whites, 1980-1988." Annals of Epidemiology 8:184-91.

Baker, D. W., M. F. Shapiro, and C. L. Schur. 2000. "Health Insurance and Access to Care for Symptomatic Conditions." Archives of Internal Medicine 160(9):1269-74.

Barker, D. J., D. Coggon, C. Osmond, and C. Wickham. 1990. "Poor Housing in Childhood and High Rates of Stomach Cancer in England and Wales." British Journal of Cancer 61(4):575-8.

Barrow, S. M., D. B. Herman, P. Cordova, and E. L. Struening. 1999. "Mortality Among Homeless Shelter Residents in New York City." American Journal of Public Health 89(4):529-34.

Beauchamp, D. 1997. "Public Health, Privatization, and Market Populism: A Time for Reflection." Quality Management in Health Care 5(2):73-9.

Berkman, L. F. 2004. "Introduction: Seeing the Forest and the Trees—From Observation to Experiments in Social Epidemiology." Epidemiologic Reviews 26:2-6.

Blakely, T. A., B. P. Kennedy, and I. Kawachi. 2001. "Socioeconomic Inequality in Voting Participation and Self-Rated Health." American Journal of Public Health 91(1):99-104.

Blindauer, K. M., R. J. Jackson, and M. McGeehin. 1999. "Environmental Pesticide Illness and Injury: The Need for a National Surveillance System." Journal of Environmental Health 61(10):9-13.

Continued on next page

Bosma, H., H. D. van de Mheen, G. J. J. M. Borsboom, and J. P. Mackenbach. 2001. "Neighborhood Socioeconomic Status and All-Cause Mortality." American Journal of Epidemiology 153(4):363-71.

Bratton, K. A., and K. L. Haynie. 1999. "Agenda Setting and Legislative Success in State Legislatures: The Effects of Gender and Race." Journal of Politics 61(3): 658-79.

Brown, P. 1995. "Race, Class, and Environmental Health: A Review and Systematization of the Literature." Environmental Research 69:15-30.

Carstairs, V., and R. Morris. 1989. "Deprivation: Explaining Differences in Mortality Between Scotland and England and Wales." British Medical Journal 299:886-9.

Cassel, J. 1976. "The Contribution of the Social Environment to Host Resistance." American Journal of Epidemiology 104(2):107-23.

Cheng, Y., I. Kawachi, E. H. Caokley, J. Schwartz, and G. Colditz. 2000. "Association Between Psychosocial Work Characteristics and Health Functioning in American Women: Prospective Study." British Medical Journal 320(7247):1432-6.

Cohen, D., S. Spear, R. Scribner, P. Kissinger, K. Mason, and J. Wildgen. 2000. "'Broken Windows' and the Risk of Gonorrhea." American Journal of Public Health 90:230-6.

Coleman, J. S. 1988. "Social Capital in the Creation of Human Capital." American Journal of Sociology 94:S95-S120.

Collins, C. A., and D. R. Williams. 1999. "Segregation and Mortality: The Deadly Effects of Racism?" Sociological Forum 14(3):495-523.

Cubbin, C., F. B. LeClere, and G. S. Smith. 2000. "Socioeconomic Status and Injury Mortality: Individual and Neighborhood Determinants." Journal of Epidemiology and Community Health 54:517-24.

Davey Smith, G., and D. Dorling. 1996. "'I'm All Right, John': Voting Patterns and Mortality in England and Wales, 1981-92." British Medical Journal 313:1573-7.

Davey Smith, G., and N. Krieger. 2004. "'Bodies Count,' and Body Counts: Social Epidemiology and Embodying Inequality." Epidemiologic Reviews 26:92-103.

Dedman, D. J., D. Gunnell, G. Davey Smith, and S. Frankel. 2001. "Childhood Housing Conditions and Later Mortality in the Boyd Orr Cohort." Journal of Epidemiology and Community Health 55(1):10-5.

de Jonge, J., H. Bosma, R. Peter, and J. Siegrist. 2000. "Job Strain, Effort-Reward Imbalance and Employee Well-Being: A Large-Scale Cross-Sectional Study." Social Science and Medicine 50:1317-27.

Continued on next page

Diez Roux, A. V. 1998. "Bringing Context Back into Epidemiology: Variables and Fallacies in Multilevel Analysis." American Journal of Public Health 88(2):216-22.

Diez Roux, A. V. 2004. "The Study of Group-Level Factors in Epidemiology: Rethinking Variables, Study Designs, and Analytical Approaches." Epidemiologic Reviews 26:104-11.

Diez Roux, A. V., F. J. Nieto, C. Muntaner, H. A. Tyroler, G. W. Comstock, E. Shahar, L. S. Cooper, R. L. Watson, and M. Szklo. 1997. "Neighborhood Environments and Coronary Heart Disease: A Multilevel Analysis." American Journal of Epidemiology 146(1):48-63.

Diez Roux, A. V., S. S. Merkin, D. Arnett, L. Chambless, M. Massing, F. J. Nieto, P. Sorlie, M. Szklo, H. A. Tyroler, and R. L. Watson. 2001. "Neighborhood of Residence and Incidence of Coronary Heart Disease." New England Journal of Medicine 345(2):99-106.

Durkin, M. S., L. L. Davidson, L. Kuhn, P. OConnor, and B. Barlow. 1994. "Low-Income Neighborhoods and the Risk of Severe Pediatric Injury: A Small-Area Analysis in Northern Manhattan." American Journal of Public Health 84(4):587-92.

Ellaway, A., and S. Macintyre. 1998. "Does Housing Tenure Predict Health in the UK Because It Exposes People to Different Levels of Housing Related Hazards in the Home or Its Surroundings?" Health and Place 4(2):141-50.

Ellaway, A., and S. Macintyre. 2000. "Mums on Prozac, Kids on Inhalers: The Need for Research on the Potential for Improving Health Through Housing Interventions." Health Bulletin 58(4):336-9.

Ferguson, T. 1995. Golden Rule: The Investment Theory of Party Competition and the Logic of Money-Driven Political Systems. Chicago: University of Chicago Press.

Filakti, H., and J. Fox. 1995. "Differences in Mortality by Housing Tenure and by Car Access from the OPCS Longitudinal Study." Population Trends 81:27-30.

Fingerhut, L. A., and M. Warner. 1997. "Health, United States, 1996-97 and Injury Chartbook." Hyattsville, MD: National Center for Health Statistics.

Flores, G., M. Abreu, M. A. Olivar, and B. Kustner. 1998. "Access Barriers to Health Care for Latino Children." Archives of Pediatric and Adolescent Medicine 152(1):1119-25.

French, S. A., M. Story, and R. W. Jeffery. 2001. "Environmental Influences on Eating and Physical Activity." Annual Review of Public Health 22:309-35.

Frenk, J. 1998. "Medical Care and Health Improvement: The Critical Link." Annals of Internal Medicine 129:419-20.

Continued on next page

Gielen, A. C., M. E. Wilson, R. R. Faden, L. Wissow, and J. D. Harvilchuck. 1995. "In-Home Injury Prevention Practices for Infants and Toddlers: The Role of Parental Beliefs, Barriers, and Housing Quality." Health Education Quarterly 22(1):85-95.

Goldman, L. R., M. W. Shannon, and the American Academy of Pediatrics Committee on Environmental Health. 2001. "Technical Report: Mercury in the Environment: Implications for Pediatricians." Pediatrics 108(1):197-205.

Greenough, G., M. McGeehin, S. M. Bernard, J. Trtanj, J. Riad, and D. Engelberg. 2001. "The Potential Impacts of Climate Variability and Change on Health Impacts of Extreme Weather Events in the United States." Environmental Health Perspectives 109(suppl 2):191-8.

Griffith, J., R. Duncan, W. Riggan, and A. Pellom. 1989. "Cancer Mortality in U.S. Counties With Hazardous Waste Sites and Ground Water Pollution" Archives of Environmental Health 44:69-74.

Grossman, D. C., H. J. Neckerman, T. D. Koepsell, P. Y. Liu, K. N. Asher, K. Beland, K. Frey, and F. P. Rivara. 1997. "Effectiveness of a Violence Prevention Curriculum Among Children in Elementary School. A Randomized Controlled Trial." Journal of the American Medical Association 77(20):1605-11.

Guest, A. M., G. Almgren, and J. M. Hussey. 1998. "The Ecology of Race and Socioeconomic Distress: Infant and Working-Age Mortality in Chicago." Demography 35(1):23-34.

Hill, K. Q., and J. E. Leighley. 1992. "The Policy Consequences of Class Bias in State Electorates." American Journal of Political Science 36(2):351-65.

Hirsch, B. T., and D. A. Macpherson. 2001. Union Membership and Earnings Data Book: Compilations from the Current Population Survey. Washington, DC: Bureau of National Affairs.

Holzer, H. 1991. "The Spatial Mismatch Hypothesis: What Has the Evidence Shown?" Urban Studies 28:105-22.

House, J. S., C. Robbins, and H. Metzner. 1982. "The Association of Social Relations and Activities with Mortality. Prospective Evidence from the Tecumseh Community Health Study." American Journal of Epidemiology 116:123-40.

House, J. S., K. R. Landis, and D. Umberson. 1988. "Social Relationships and Health." Science 241:540-5.

Howell E. M., K. L. Pettit, B. A. Ormond, and G. T. Kingsley. 2003. "Using the National Neighborhood Indicators Partnership to Improve Public Health." Journal of Public Health Management Practice 9(3):235-42.

Hwang, S. W. 2001. "Homelessness and Health." Canadian Medical Association Journal 164(2):229-33.

Institute of Medicine. 1988. The Future of Public Health. Washington, DC: National Academy Press.

Continued on next page

Institute of Medicine. 1993. Access to Health Care in America. Washington, DC: National Academy Press.

Institute of Medicine. 1997. Improving Health in the Community: A Role for Performance Monitoring. Washington, DC: National Academy Press.

Jackson, S. A., R. T. Anderson, R. J. Johnson, and P. D. Sorlie. 2000. "The Relation of Residential Segregation to All-Cause Mortality: A Study in Black and White." American Journal of Public Health 90(4):615-7.

Johnson, B. L. 1999. "A Review of the Effects of Hazardous Waste on Reproductive Health." American Journal of Obstetrics and Gynecology 181(1):12-6.

Kaplan, G. A., and J. W. Lynch. 1997. "Whither Studies on the Socioeconomic Foundations of Population Health?" American Journal of Public Health 87(9):1409-11.

Kaplan, G. A., and J. W. Lynch. 2001. "Is Economic Policy Health Policy?" American Journal of Public Health 91(3):1-3.

Kawachi, I. 1999. "Social Capital and Community Effects on Population and Individual Health." Annals of the New York Academy of Sciences 896:120-30.

Kawachi, I., B. P. Kennedy, K. Lochner, and D. Prothrow-Stith. 1997. "Social Capital, Income Inequality, and Mortality." American Journal of Public Health 87(9):1491-8.

Kawachi, I., B. P. Kennedy, and R. Glass. 1999a. "Social Capital and Self-Rated Health: A Contextual Analysis." American Journal of Public Health 89:1187-93.

Kawachi, I., B. P. Kennedy, and R. G. Wilkinson. 1999b. "Crime: Social Disorganization and Relative Deprivation." Social Science and Medicine 48:719-31.

Kennedy, B. P., I. Kawachi, R. Glass, and D. Prothrow-Stith D. 1998. "Income Distribution, Socioeconomic Status, and Self Rated Health in the United States: Multilevel Analysis." British Medical Journal 317:917-21.

Ketola, E., R. Sipila, and M. Makela. 2000. "Effectiveness of Individual Lifestyle Interventions in Reducing Cardiovascular Disease and Risk Factors." Annals of Medicine 32(4):239-51.

Krieger, N., J. T. Chen, P. D. Waterman, M. J. Soobader, S. V. Subramanian, and R. Carson. 2002. "Geocoding and Monitoring of U.S. Socioeconomic Inequalities in Mortality and Cancer Incidence: Does the Choice of Area-Based Measure and Geographic Level Matter?: The Public Health Disparities Geocoding Project." American Journal of Epidemiology 156(5):471-82.

Continued on next page

Krieger, N., J. T. Chen, P. D. Waterman, M. J. Soobader, S. V. Subramanian, and R. Carson. 2003. "Choosing Area Based Socioeconomic Measures to Monitor Social Inequalities in Low Birth Weight and Childhood Lead Poisoning: The Public Health Disparities Geocoding Project." Journal of Epidemiology and Community Health 57(3):186-99.

Krieger, N., D. L. Rowley, A. A. Herman, B. Avery, and M. T. Phillips. 1993. "Racism, Sexism and Social Class: Implications for Studies of Health, Disease, and Well-Being." American Journal of Preventive Medicine 9(suppl 2):82-122.

Krieger, N., and S. Sidney. 1997. "Prevalence and Health Implications of Anti-Gay Discrimination: A Study of Black and White Women and Men in the CARDIA Cohort." International Journal of Health Services 27(1):157-76.

Landrigan, P. J., L. Claudio, S. B. Markowitz, G. S. Berkowitz, B. L. Brenner, H. Romero, J. G. Wetmur, T. D. Matte, A. C. Gore, J. H. Godbold, and M. S. Wolff. 1999. "Pesticides and Inner-City Children: Exposures, Risks, and Prevention." Environmental Health Perspectives 107(suppl 3):431-7.

Langer, N. 1999. "Culturally Competent Professionals in Therapeutic Alliances Enhance Patient Compliance." Journal of Health Care for the Poor and Underserved 10(1):19-26.

LeClere, F. B., R. G. Rogers, and K. D. Peters. 1998. "Neighborhood Social Context and Racial Differences in Women's Heart Disease Mortality." Journal of Health Social Behavior 39:91-107.

Lynch, J. W., and G. A. Kaplan. 2000. "Socioeconomic Position." In Social Epidemiology, edited by L. F. Berkman and I. Kawachi, 13-35. New York: Oxford University Press.

Lynch, J. W., G. A. Kaplan, E. R. Pamuk, R. D. Cohen, K. E. Heck, J. L. Balfour, and I. H. Yen. 1998. "Income Inequality and Mortality in Metropolitan Areas of the United States." American Journal of Public Health 88(7):1074-80.

Lynch, J. W., P. Due, C. Muntaner, and G. Davey Smith. 2000b. "Social Capital—Is It a Good Strategy for Public Health?" Journal of Epidemiology and Community Health 54:404-8.

Macintyre, S., A. Ellaway, G. Der, G. Ford, and K. Hunt. 1998. "Do Housing Tenure and Car Access Predict Health Because They are Simply Markers of Income or Self Esteem? A Scottish Study." Journal of Epidemiology and Community Health 52:657-64.

Macintyre, S., A. Ellaway, and S. Cummins. 2002. "Place Effects on Health: How Can We Conceptualise, Operationalise and Measure Them?" Social Science and Medicine 55:125-39.

McGinnis, M. J., and W. H. Foege. 1998. "Actual Causes of Death in the United States." Journal of the American Medical Association 270:2207-12.

Continued on next page

McKeown, T. 1979. The Role of Medicine: Dream, Mirage, or Nemesis? Princeton, NJ: Princeton University Press.

McQuiston, T. H., R. C. Zakocs, and D. Loomis. 1998. "The Case for Stronger OSHA Enforcement—Evidence From Evaluation Research." American Journal of Public Health 88(7):1022-4.

Mendelsohn, A. L., B. P. Dreyer, A. H. Fierman, C. M. Rosen, L. A. Legano, H. A. Kruger, S. W. Lim, S. Barasch, L. Au, and C. D. Courtlandt. 1999. "Low-Level Lead Exposure and Cognitive Development in Early Childhood." Journal of Developmental and Behavioral Pediatrics 20(6):425-31.

Miringoff, M., and M-L. Miringoff. 1999. The Social Health of the Nation. New York: Oxford University Press.

Mitchell, R., S. Gleave, M. Bartley, D. Wiggins, and H. Joshi. 2000. "Do Attitude and Area Influence Health? A Multilevel Approach to Health Inequalities." Health and Place 6:67-79.

Mitchell-Weaver, C., D. Miller, and R. Deal. 2000. "Municipal Governance and Metropolitan Regionalism in the USA." Urban Studies 37(516):851-76.

Mouw, T. 2000. "Job Relocation and the Racial Gap in Unemployment in Detroit and Chicago, 1980 to 1990." American Sociological Review 65:730-53.

Nansel, T. R., M. Overpeck, R. S. Pilla, W. J. Ruan, B. Simons-Morton, and P. Scheidt. 2001. "Bullying Behaviors Among U.S. Youth: Prevalence and Association With Psychosocial Adjustment." Journal of the American Medical Association 285(16):2094-100.

Navin, F., S. Zein, and E. Felipe. 2000. "Road Safety Engineering: An Effective Tool in the Fight Against Whiplash Injuries." Accident Analysis and Prevention 32(2):271-5.

Nelson, D. E., B. L. Thompson, S. D. Bland, and R. Rubinson. 1999. "Trends in Perceived Cost as a Barrier to Medical Care, 1991-1996." American Journal of Public Health 89(9):1410-3.

Newacheck, P. W., J. J. Stoddard, D. C. Hughes, and M. Pearl. 1998. "Health Insurance and Access to Primary Care for Children." New England Journal of Medicine 338:513-9.

O'Campo, P., X. Xue, M.-C. Wang, and M. O. Caughy. 1997. "Neighborhood Risk Factors for Low Birthweight in Baltimore: A Multilevel Analysis." American Journal of Public Health 87(7):1113-8.

Packer, C. N., S. Stewart-Brown, and S. E. Fowle. 1994. "Damp Housing and Adult Health: Results From a Lifestyle Study in Worcester, England." Journal of Epidemiology and Community Health 48:555-9.

Passchier-Vermeer, W., and W. F. Passchier. 2000. "Noise Exposure and Public Health." Environmental Health Perspectives 108(suppl 1):123-31.

Continued on next page

Patz, J. A., M. A. McGeehin, and S. M. Bernard. 2001. "The Potential Health Impacts of Climate Variability and Change for the United States." Journal of Environmental Health 64(2):20-8.

Pickett, K. E., and M. Pearl. 2001. "Multilevel Analyses of Neighbourhood Socioeconomic Context and Health Outcomes: A Critical Review." Journal of Epidemiology and Community Health 55:111-22.

Pincus, T., R. Esther, D. A. DeWalt, and L. F. Callahan. 1998. "Social Conditions and Self-Management Are More Powerful Determinants of Health Than Access to Care." Annals of Internal Medicine 129:406-11.

Platt, S., C. Martin, S. Hunt, and C. Lewis. 1989. "Damp Housing, Mould Growth and Symptomatic Health State." British Medical Journal 298:1643-8.

Pope, C. A. 3rd, D. V. Bates, and M. E. Raizenne. 1995. "Health Effects of Particulate Air Pollution: Time for Reassessment?" Environmental Health Perspectives 103(5):472-80.

Portes, A. 1998. "Social Capital: Its Origins and Applications to Modern Sociology." American Journal of Sociology 24:1-24.

Pugh, M. 1998. Barriers to Work: The Spatial Divide Between Jobs and Welfare Recipients in Metropolitan Areas. Brookings Institution Center on Urban and Metropolitan Policy. Available at http://www.brookings.edu/es/urban/mismatch.pdf.

Putnam, R., R. Leonardi, and R. Nanetti. 1993. Making Democracy Work: Civic Traditions in Modern Italy. Princeton, NJ: Princeton University Press.

Roberts, E. M. 1997. "Neighborhood Social Environments and the Distribution of Low Birthweight in Chicago." American Journal of Public Health 87(4):597-603.

Ross, B. H, and M. A. Levine. 1996. Urban Politics: Power in Metropolitan America. 5th edition. N. Itasca, IL: FE Peacock.

Saltzstein, A. L., Y. Ting, and G. H. Saltzstein. 2001. "Work-Family Balance and Job Satisfaction: The Impact of Family-Friendly Policies on Attitudes of Federal Government Employees." Public Administration Review 61(4):452-67.

Sampson, R. J., S. W. Raudenbush, and F. Earls. 1997. "Neighborhoods and Violent Crime: A Multilevel Study of Collective Efficacy." Science 277:918-24.

Schell, L. M. 1991. "Effects of Pollutants on Human Prenatal and Postnatal Growth: Noise, Lead, Polychlorobiphenyl Compounds, and Toxic Wastes." American Journal of Physical Anthropology (suppl 13):157-88.

Schoenbach, V. J., B. H. Kaplan, L. Fredman, and D. G. Kleinbaum. 1986. "Social Ties and Mortality in Evans County, Georgia." American Journal of Epidemiology 123:577-91.

Continued on next page

Sharpe, M. 1999. "An Unhealthy Road." Journal of Environmental Monitoring 1:23N-25N.

Shaw, M., D. Gordon, D. Dorling, R. Mitchell, and G. Davey Smith. 2000. "Increasing Mortality Differentials by Residential Area Level of Poverty: Britain 1981-1997." Social Science and Medicine 51:151-3.

Snyder, P., J. Anliker, L. Cunningham-Sabo, L. B. Dixon, J. Altaha, A. Chamberlain, S. Davis, M. Evans, J. Hurley, and J. L. Weber. 1999. "The Pathways Study: A Model For Lowering the Fat in School Meals." American Journal of Clinical Nutrition 69(4 suppl):810S-815S.

Stone, E. J., T. L. McKenzie, G. J. Welk, and M. L. Booth. 1998. "Effects of Physical Activity Interventions in Youth: Review and Synthesis." American Journal of Preventive Medicine 15(4):298-315.

Styne, D. M. 2001. "Childhood and Adolescent Obesity: Prevalence and Significance." Pediatric Clinics of North America 48(4):823-54.

Subramanian, S.V., I. Kawachi, and B. P. Kennedy. 2001. "Does the State You Live In Make a Difference? Multilevel Analysis of Self-Rated Health in the US." Social Science and Medicine 53:9-19.

Susser, M., W. Watson, and K. Hopper. 1985. Sociology in Medicine. New York: Oxford University Press.

Townsend, P., P. Phillimore, and A. Beattie. 1988. Health and Deprivation: Inequality and the North. London: Croom Helm.

Turnlock, B. J., and A. S. Handler. 1997. "From Measuring to Improving Public Health Practice." Annual Review of Public Health 18:261-82.

Twemlow, S. W., P. Fonagy, F. C. Sacco, M. L. Gies, R. Evans, and R. Ewbank. 2001. "Creating a Peaceful School Learning Environment: A Controlled Study of an Elementary School Intervention to Reduce Violence." American Journal of Psychiatry 158(5):808-10.

U. S. Department of Health and Human Services (USDHHS). 2000. Healthy People 2010. Washington, DC: U. S. Department of Health and Human Services.

U. S. Preventive Services Task Force. 1996. Guide to Clinical Preventive Services, 2nd edition. Baltimore: Williams & Wilkins.

Waitzman, R. J., and K. R. Smith. 1998a. "Separate But Lethal: The Effects of Economic Segregation on Mortality in Metropolitan America." Milbank Memorial Quarterly 76(3):341-73.

Waitzman, R. J., and K. R. Smith. 1998b. "Phantom of the Poverty Area: Poverty-Area Residence and Mortality in the United States." American Journal of Public Health 88:973-6.

Continued on next page

Wasserman, C. R., G. M. Shaw, S. Selvin, J. B. Gould, and S. L. Syme. 1998. "Socioeconomic Status, Neighborhood Social Conditions, and Neural Tube Defects." American Journal of Public Health 88(11):1674-80.

Whitby, K. J. 1997. The Color of Representation: Congressional Behavior and Black Interests. Ann Arbor: University of Michigan Press.

Williams, D. R. 1999. "Race, Socioeconomic Status, and Health: The Added Effects of Racism and Discrimination." Annals of the New York Academy of Sciences 896:173-88.

Williams, D. R., and C. Collins. 2001. "Racial Residential Segregation: A Fundamental Cause of Racial Disparities in Health." Public Health Reports 116:404-16.

Wilson, P. S. 1994. "Established Risk Factors and Coronary Artery Disease: The Framingham Study." American Journal of Hypertension 7(pt 2):75-125.

Woolcock, M. 2001. "The Place of Social Capital in Understanding Social and Economic Outcomes." ISUMA: Canadian Journal of Policy Research 2(1):11-7.

Yen, I. H., and G. A. Kaplan. 1999. "Poverty Area Residence and Changes in Depression and Perceived Health Status: Evidence From the Alameda County Study." International Journal of Epidemiology 28:90-4.

Yen, I. H., and S. L. Syme. 1999. "The Social Environment and Health: A Discussion of the Epidemiologic Literature." Annual Review of Public Health 20:287-308.

Yen, I. H., D. R. Ragland, B. A. Greiner, and J. M. Fisher. 1999. "Workplace Discrimination and Alcohol Consumption: Findings From the San Francisco Muni Health and Safety Study." Ethnicity and Disease 9(1):70-80.

www.ingramcontent.com/pod-product-compliance
Lightning Source LLC
Chambersburg PA
CBHW081843170526
45167CB00007B/2888

* 9 7 8 1 4 9 9 5 4 9 3 7 9 *